the mothercare guide to

HEALTH, BEAUTY
≈ AND EXERCISE ≈

for pregnancy and after

the mothercare guide to

HEALTH, BEAUTY
≈ *AND EXERCISE* ≈

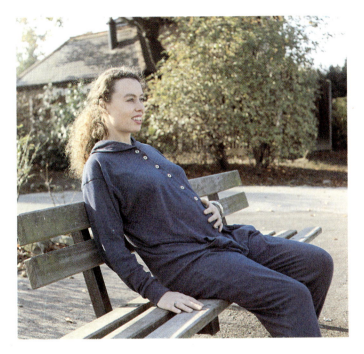

for pregnancy and after

ELISABETH MORSE

Conran Octopus

CONTENTS

Introduction   6

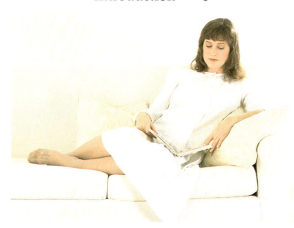

Looking after yourself   8

Your emotional approach   10   Your pregnancy wardrobe   34
Your relationships   16   Your diet   42
Your beauty routine   22   Your job   52

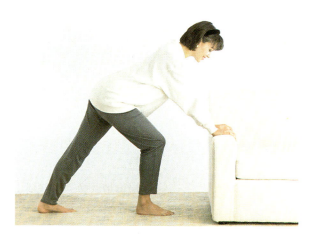

Keeping fit   58

Everyday action   60   Exercise   74
Sport and leisure   68

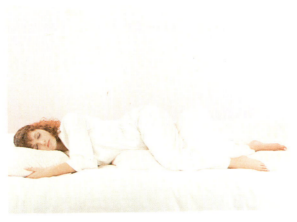

Relaxation 88

Learning to unwind 90   Massage 98

The medical background 110

Your medical care 112   Common complaints in
Your progress through   pregnancy and childbirth 118
  pregnancy 114   Glossary 122

Index 125   Acknowledgments 128

Project editor
Jane O'Shea

Art editor
Jenny Kirby

Editors
Mary Davies
Christine Mills

Project assistant
Denise Bates

Picture research
Nadine Bazar

Production
Shane Lask

First published in 1989 by
Conran Octopus Limited
37 Shelton Street
London WC2H 9HN

Text copyright © 1989 Elisabeth Morse
Artwork copyright © 1989 Conran Octopus

ISBN 1 85029 210 8

Typeset by Bookworm Typesetting, Manchester
Printed in Spain by Novograph, S.A.

INTRODUCTION

*P*regnancy is a normal experience for the majority of women. However, normal never means simply ordinary. To you, it will probably feel quite extraordinary, whether you love being pregnant or whether you don't.

Pregnancy brings all sorts of changes which can be fascinating or irritating. Either way you are likely to find that you become more and more involved with yourself and your 'bump'. But you will also be thinking more about your relationships with other people – your partner, your mother, your brothers and sisters, the rest of your family and your friends – whether this is your first child or not.

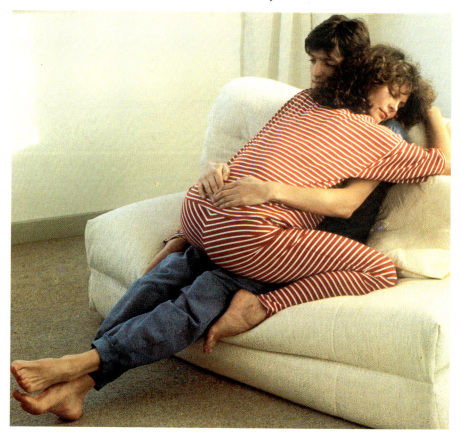

You prepare mentally as well as physically for the birth of a baby. How much you choose to grow mentally and emotionally during your pregnancy – using the time to adjust and adapt – is up to you. But, if you let it, pregnancy can offer a unique opportunity to get to know your strengths and your capabilities better. Getting to know yourself is not the same as becoming totally self-centred. Rather it is an important part of building the reserves of confidence and understanding we all need to cope with any big change in life.

The welfare and happiness of a mother and her child are inextricably linked in the early weeks and months of a baby's life. In the best relationships there is a delicate balance of give and take. The woman who has decided to give herself over completely to the care of her baby risks the happiness of them both just as surely as the woman who is determined not to let her baby interfere with her life.

This book tells you all about the changes that are likely to happen during pregnancy and the early months after the birth, so that you can decide how you can make the most of them. It is also about sharing the good and the bad with your partner and with other women so that by listening and learning from each other you build up a network of mutual support. In these ways pregnancy need not be a limbo time while you simply wait for the birth. It can be an enriching and rewarding opportunity for you to build on your understanding and resourcefulness so that you can meet with confidence the many challenges that will face you as a parent.

Shaping your future
Throughout the book many suggestions are made for ways of taking care of yourself. They have been developed from the combined expertise of experienced mothers, as well as doctors and others with specialist skills. Most of the theories have been tried out in practice and modified by experience. Some of the ideas may be familiar and some will be new. Some of the suggestions will suit you and others won't. If you use your pregnancy to try out new approaches and rethink old ones, the experience will open up fresh possibilities rather than shut the door on past freedoms. All the exercises, relaxation techniques and fitness routines are based on fundamental principles which will be of value to you for the rest of your life.

LOOKING AFTER YOURSELF

Pregnancy provides an opportunity to get to know yourself through the changes you will experience. Benefit from giving yourself extra care and attention and your increased self-esteem will help you adapt after your baby is born.

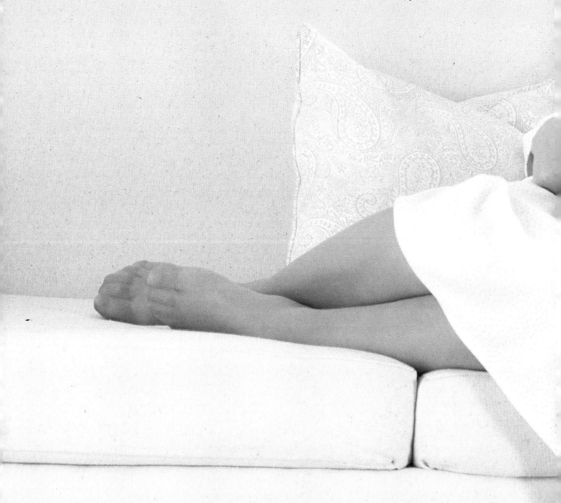

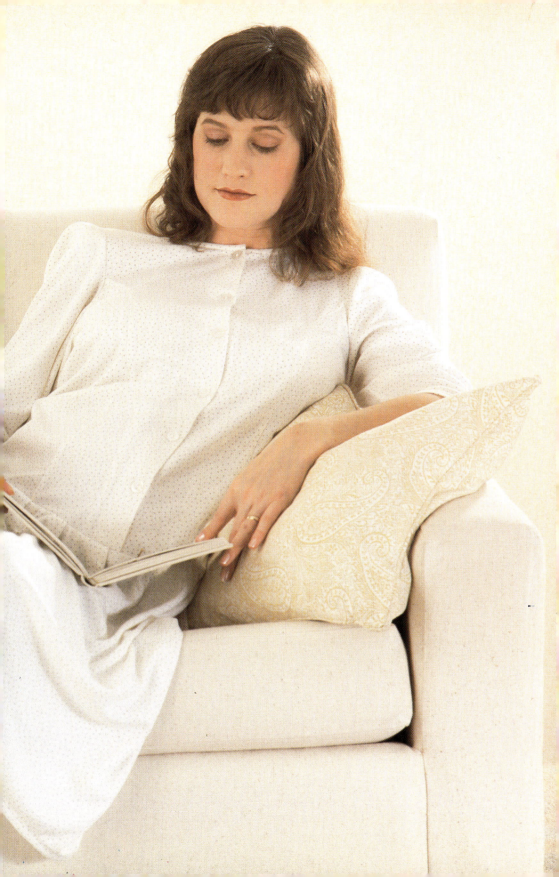

YOUR EMOTIONAL
≈ *APPROACH* ≈

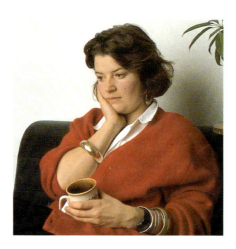

*I*n the first three or four months of pregnancy you are more likely to be preoccupied with the idea of *being* pregnant than with living up to the traditional image of the 'radiant, serene' mother-to-be!

Whether the event is planned or unplanned, getting a positive result to a pregnancy test often produces a mixture of feelings. Initial excitement or dismay can give way to disbelief, pride that you are able to conceive, apprehension because life will never be the same again, worry because you had too many drinks at a party the week before, awe at the amazing process which has begun within your body and joy because you are setting out on a new adventure. And, with the early months such a critical stage in the development of your baby, you may also be overwhelmed by a sense of responsibility as well as fears that you could miscarry. Equally, the early weeks can seem a limbo. You don't look pregnant yet you have to handle the reactions and emotions of family and friends, and you must decide where you are going to have your baby.

Telling people you are pregnant can have unexpected repercussions too. Your pregnancy, which started as a very private matter between you and your partner, can rapidly become a very public concern. You may welcome the attention or you may feel uncomfortable about this apparent intrusion or you may feel both.

All these feelings are not only normal, they actually help you cope successfully with the inevitable changes which will happen to you, your life and your relationships.

As part of the process of facing up to change, you may find yourself going over past experiences and relationships. This may seem strange but it springs from a psychological need to check out exactly where you are at this point in your life before you embark on the next stage.

Pregnancy is one of those life-events which offer you an opportunity to get to know yourself better. On bad days – and there will be some – it will help if you find something pleasurable to compensate, whether it be curling up with a good book or treating yourself to a beauty treatment. Giving yourself some care is not vain self-indulgence but can be a very good way of learning to do the same for others, not least the baby growing inside you.

The middle months
By the fourth and fifth months, when you have had a thorough medical check-up at the antenatal clinic, you will probably be feeling much more confident. Your bump will be starting to show but not so much that you cannot hide it when you want to. You may take a real pleasure in your rounded shape and, if your skin and hair have improved, you will be feeling much more positive.

Feeling your baby move – at first like a fluttering, and later an unmistakeable kicking – is uniquely exciting. You may find the fact you cannot control your baby's movements which are, after all, a part of your body quite remarkable, if not weird. You will become spellbound from time to time as you wonder just what causes these spurts of activity. And you may well talk to your bump as if it were another person. This growing fascination and wonder as you try and imagine the baby inside you is all part of preparing yourself for the existence of another person in your life.

'I'm fed up with everyone saying, "You've done it now. Life won't ever be the same again." I want to enjoy my pregnancy. Not have it spoilt.'

11

The role of anxiety

*I*t is quite common for the first-time mother in particular to worry about *being worried*. You may feel obsessed with every alteration in your appearance. You may fear being 'boring' about every new development in your baby. You may wonder about your sense of proportion when remarks like 'that baby's going to be a handful judging from the activity in your tum' fill you with apprehension. And you may doubt your reason as you weep over 'silly' things.

Any big change in life causes anxiety. A certain amount of anxiety is healthy. It puts us 'on our mettle', ready for any problems that may arise and able mentally to rehearse every likely experience so that we can plan how to deal with it. Used positively, anxiety can help us become more open and more realistic.

When you are pregnant, anxiety is a very important way not only of preparing and coming to terms with your future responsibilities but also of alerting you to any changes which may be significant. You are already beginning to adjust to caring for your new baby and that means being ready to ward off possible dangers. 'Don't worry' is therefore unhelpful, and often impossible, advice to follow.

Preparing for parenthood
Much of your mental preparation takes place subconsciously. You may simply be aware of ups and downs as vague unease alternates with excitement. Some psychologists believe that this is the cause of the vivid dreams which pregnant women often have.

Over-anxiety, on the other hand, is no help. It can exhaust you, it may make you want to run away rather than face up to a problem or it may simply paralyze you completely. Talking over your worries with someone who will listen nearly always helps; so does making an effort to find out how real your fear is. Discussion with someone who has your interests at heart will usually show you that your problem is not as bad as you had imagined. If anxiety keeps you awake at night, keep a notepad by your bed and write your fears down – and the reasons for them. This often helps to put them into perspective.

Don't envy the apparently carefree mother-to-be. If being carefree means that no adjustments have been made in advance, then the realities of birth and the new baby can be a huge shock. True confidence comes from working *through* anxieties to gain an understanding of your own strengths and limitations.

'Pregnancy has made me feel closer to other women. I've discovered a deeper respect for them – and myself.'

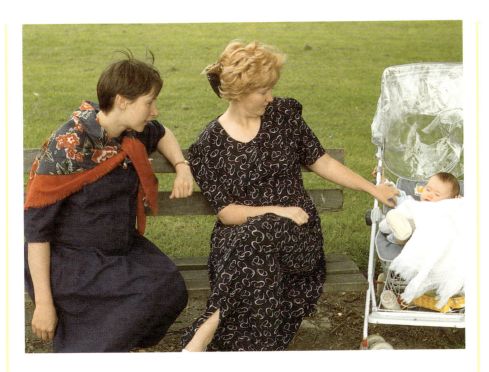

Later pregnancy

*H*owever excited or resentful you may have been when you first discovered you were pregnant, by the end of the sixth month your attitude may well be ambivalent. You will be both looking forward to the birth and somewhat apprehensive. In the last two or three months, as the time draws nearer and the realization that your bump will produce a baby really begins to dawn, anxieties may surface again. Antenatal classes, if you attend them, are likely to start sometime during the seventh month and this can make the actual fact of labour even more of a reality – something which you may or may not find very welcome.

Towards the end of pregnancy you may find your bump feels too much to cope with and your patience can wear thin. The baby may be pushing on your lungs, making breathing difficult, or pressing on your bladder; and you may be feeling more contractions – even finding some of them unexpectedly painful.

Giving up work may be a relief or yet another unwelcome reminder that life is changing. You may ask yourself why you should have to go through all this *and* a probably painful labour. On the other hand, you will be meeting other pregnant women, at the antenatal clinic or at classes, making what could be lifelong friends.

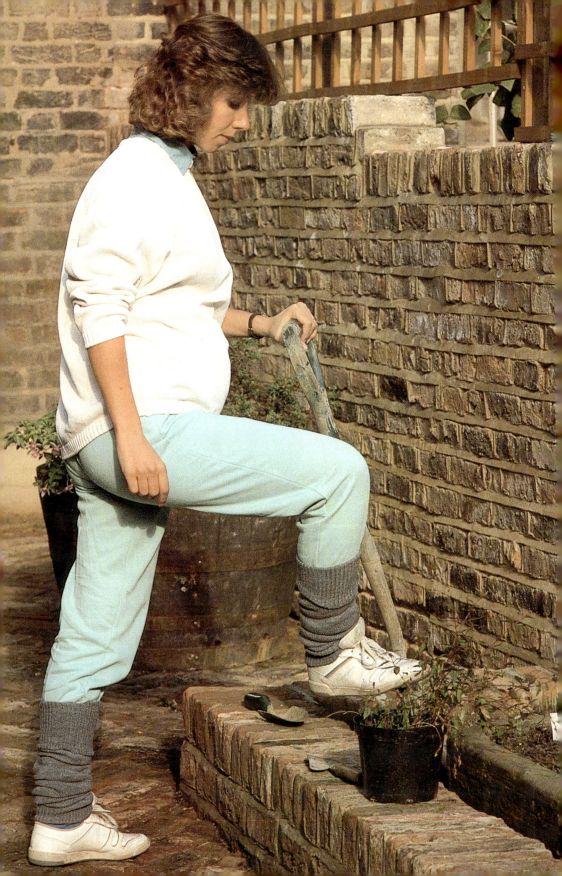

Myths about motherhood

*T*wo of the most common myths you may hear during pregnancy are that you will love your baby instantly and that motherhood is instinctive. Both can cause great anxiety for any mother-to-be.

It is a very common and normal reaction to fear that you will not love your baby. It can strike while you are pregnant or after the baby is born. If you were to believe all the advertisements you see, you'd think that loving a baby is automatic; it can be hard to acknowledge your misgivings if you fear you are the only one thinking that way.

There is no reason why you should fall automatically in love with your new baby. One of the most extraordinary things about seeing your baby for the first time is the acute awareness that this is *another person* – not some living doll. As with any new person in your life, you may form a loving attachment straightaway or it may take time. And your baby will react the same way. What he wants is warmth, food, somewhere to sleep and to be held. Love is doing things for someone else, not just an overwhelming feeling in your heart. Love also has an endless capacity to grow so it is possible to be 'in love' with more than one child at once – sometimes hard to believe with a second baby on the way.

Equally, there is no need to fear that you lack the instincts of true motherhood. Knowing how to look after your baby is a skill which is learned. It has more to do with common sense than with either instinct or the theories of 'experts'. Human beings learn how to look after their babies by watching others. The learning process will have started when you were a child and watched your mother and other mothers looking after their children.

But parents probably learn most from the mistakes they make themselves, and this is true even of those expecting their third or fourth child. Every child is different and each has his own needs. Children can be both very affectionate and very hurtful, kind and unkind, cooperative and rebellious. Because the relationship between a parent and child is so intense it can bring out negative feelings in the parent too. This can be a shock if you aren't aware that it can, and does, happen to most people.

The important thing is to forgive yourself when things go wrong. Say you are sorry if need be and comfort yourself with the thought that a 'perfect' parent would be an awful burden to your child. He would probably feel that being 'perfect' was essential to being loved.

'Why didn't my friends tell me what it would be like? It's only now they ask if I'm sleeping and are my nipples sore.'

15

YOUR
≈ *RELATIONSHIPS* ≈

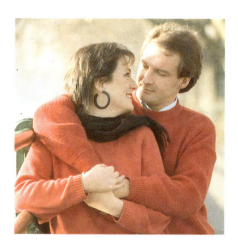

*A*lthough the baby is growing inside you, that process has its effect on everyone you know. The person quite naturally most affected is your partner. It can be a particularly difficult time for men, who are often not used to discussing their feelings, except with their partners. If you are preoccupied or confused, you may be looking to him for support rather than being able to give him the friendship he needs.

Your partner's feelings

Fathers-to-be can feel quite ambivalent during pregnancy. They may be apprehensive, either about highly practical matters, like making do with less money at a time when expenses are bound to increase, or with more emotional concerns, like what does it actually mean to be a father. They will probably also be enthusiastic and plain excited.

Men may also feel that they are expected to know how to look after their partners when they become mothers. A new father could be forgiven for believing he is needed only for his shoulder to cry on and his hands to make tea for an army of visitors. He may also feel he is expected to guide his partner through pregnancy and birth. It's not surprising then, if they fear they may be landed with all the responsibility and few of the pleasures, that men can view father-hood with trepidation and resentment.

You may also be experiencing a love–hate relationship during pregnancy. You may want your partner to take the lead and yet loathe the idea of him telling you what to do. It will help if you can both remind yourselves that as future parents you are *partners* with different experiences and different areas of expertise. The more you can share, the more support you will be able to give each other.

One of the best ways of dispelling apprehension and tension is laughter. Placing a piece of paper on your tummy and watching the baby kick it off or trying to guess what it is up to from the bumps and lumps which appear through your abdomen can be an endless source of intrigue.

Togetherness
You may both find you have an increased need for the reassurance and comfort of just holding each other during pregnancy. For many couples, holding each other often leads to intercourse so you may need to learn that just having a cuddle is a nice thing to do.

But pregnancy and parenthood should not be expected to create an inseparable and exclusive bond between the two of you. You will both need other people for support and friendship and to take the pressures off each other at what could be a difficult time.

If you have friends who are also expecting babies, it is worth making an effort to spend more time with them. Your mutual support will help you realize how much you have already learned and experienced – good for both your confidence and morale. Going to antenatal classes for couples can be a useful way of meeting other people in the same position as yourselves.

When men do allow themselves to talk with other men about their feelings and experiences, they often find it more helpful than they expected. Hearing other men's experience with in-laws who have just become grandparents, with toddlers who've acquired a baby brother or sister or with partners who may be moody and temperamental is often very helpful.

'It's incredible watching the baby kicking inside her – to think we did that!'

Within the family

You and your partner are not the only ones who have to adjust to change. A pregnancy has repercussions on the rest of the family too. Becoming a grandparent for the first time can produce an unexpected mixture of feelings.

A grandfather may be delighted about becoming a grandparent but less sure of the pleasures of being married to a grandmother! A prospective grandmother may be more involved when her daughter is expecting a baby than when her son is. She may want to relive her early days as a mother – and try persuading you to handle the experience the way she did – or she may surprise herself by resenting the new baby because it is disturbing *her* baby's sleep. And, if her children have only recently left home, she may fear being expected to become a permanently available babysitter.

Grandparents may not always offer the support you hoped for and you may have to think carefully about these relationships both before and after the birth. How, for instance, are you going to tackle implied criticism or make the most of offers of help?

'The week the three of us had together at home gave
John and me a wonderful start getting to know our new baby.'

Other children
When it comes to preparing a toddler, there is probably no way of preventing jealousy. He is bound to feel some worry because he is no longer the centre of attention as 'your baby'. Reassurance that you won't love him any less just because he has a new brother or sister is essential. It's probably more helpful to plan how to cope with jealousy attacks when they do arise. The list opposite indicates some of the ways parents have tried to prepare a young child before and after the arrival of a new baby.

Older children may need reassurance too, but obviously it is easier to discuss such feelings when the children are more mature. How well brothers and sisters eventually get on will depend as much on their personalities as anything else.

Children need the reassurance that they are loved through all the changes in their lives brought about by growing up, whether the reason is a new baby, being potty trained, learning to share with others, starting play school or moving house. So, if your toddler does become more bad-tempered, aggressive or clingy while you are pregnant, it may not be just because another baby is on the way.

'Baby drew on the wall, not me.'

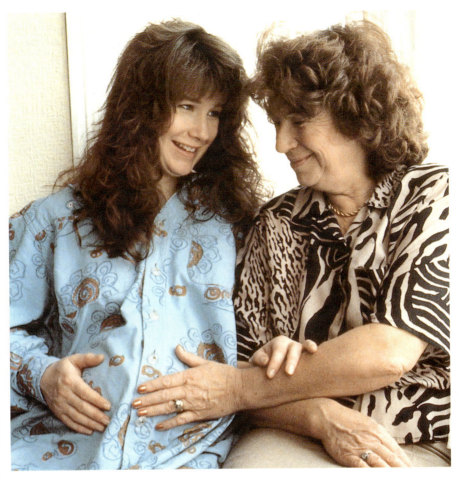

Preparing toddlers for the new baby

☐ Do antenatal exercises with him so that he helps you prepare for the baby.

☐ Show him pictures of himself as a baby and discuss how he changed as he grew up.

☐ Give him some food and a drink when he comes to visit you in hospital.

☐ Show him how he can help with the baby: getting nappies, stroking her and helping to bath her. But make sure the baby is close at hand so that you can always get to her first before he tries to lift her up.

☐ Give him a doll so he can be a Mummy or Daddy too.

☐ Read him stories about children who found new babies boring and 'in the way' and how they got used to them.

☐ Don't criticize him for disliking the baby and only intervene if the baby is likely to get hurt.

☐ Tell him the baby is looking at him and is very interested in what he is doing and saying.

Gaining confidence in yourself

*M*any women are not very good at asserting themselves. They allow themselves to be taken advantage of; they underestimate their own capabilities while overestimating other people's; they bottle up emotions and then overreact when people fail to read their minds; they label themselves 'stupid' but aren't tolerant of others' mistakes; and they want always to be liked and 'do the right thing'.

These are all symptoms of a lack of self confidence. People who have difficulty valuing themselves usually behave in one of three ways: they can be aggressive, submissive or highly manipulative. We all reveal these personality traits at times, particularly when we are anxious or feeling vulnerable.

Pregnancy can be both a boost to confidence and a time when reassurance is desperately needed. When you are confident, you gain self-respect and tolerance for others, but when you are insecure you can find it difficult to trust yourself or anyone else. These ups and downs are particularly common at the beginning and end of pregnancy, during labour and in the early weeks of parenthood.

Protecting your welfare

Learning to be assertive means expecting and giving respect to yourself and others, asking questions so that you can make decisions, and taking responsibility for yourself. It's harder in some situations than others. Asking a stranger to open a door for you is probably easier than asking your mother-in-law not to keep telling you her babies were never any trouble. And it may be easier to ask questions of a young, female health visitor in your own home than an older, male, white-coated doctor in a hospital. But asking questions and telling people how you feel is not only your privilege, it can be an important way of protecting both your own and your baby's welfare.

Asking questions helps you gain a better understanding of a situation and also gives the people who have to answer you a chance to rethink what they are saying and perhaps change their minds. Think of a situation when you were asked to explain something you wanted to do. While you set out the reasons for your point of view, didn't you find you were thinking up other, maybe more acceptable, alternatives? True discussion, when both sides contribute equally, makes it possible for the pros and cons of a situation to be weighed and often a more appropriate solution emerges.

In the case of antenatal appointments, it may help if you write down your questions beforehand and in the order in which you want to ask them. Also make a note to ask what are the possible drawbacks to any recommended course of action. In nearly every situation there

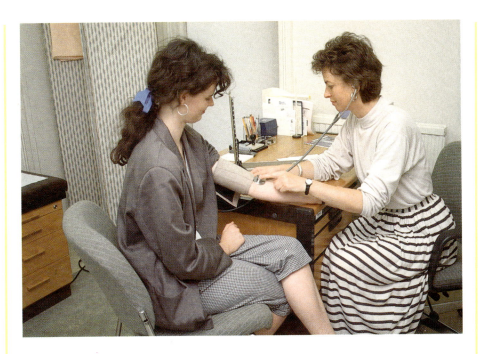

are alternative ways of treating a problem, but it's only by discussion that you can find out what the choices are and what each involves. Then you are in a position to work out between you which alternative is most appropriate for you. And, if something unexpected comes up, you can usually ask for time to think about it.

Asking questions, making yourself understood and listening to another person's point of view are not easy but these are skills which can be learned. With hindsight many mothers rate them highly. One of the commonest pieces of advice which new mothers pass on to pregnant women is 'Don't be afraid to ask questions'.

It can also help to discuss any advice you receive with people in a similar situation. Discussing 'expert' opinions with other new and prospective parents can be a useful way of working out what will suit you and your baby.

Lastly, we all need a boost to our confidence from time to time. It greatly helps relationships if you can tell others what you find helpful or have appreciated them doing for you, even if it is only to thank them for their interest.

> *'I asked the doctor if there was any medical need to induce me. She thought about it and said she'd suggested it because she thought I was tired of waiting. We talked about it and agreed it was not a good enough reason so I went home.'*

YOUR BEAUTY
≈ *ROUTINE* ≈

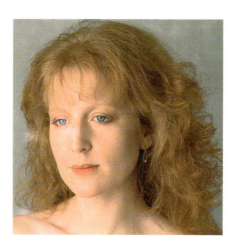

Knowing that you are looking good will usually make you feel good as well. An air of confidence and a smile on your face can make you look attractive. If pregnancy is making you bloom, as it is traditionally supposed to do, this isn't difficult. But if you are feeling sick or just fat it is much harder to look your best. Whether you feel good or not, spending time on your appearance and giving yourself some care and attention will make you feel better. It's not an indulgence but an important way of gaining confidence.

Beauty care does not simply mean carefully applied make-up and beautifully manicured nails. Not all women want to express their femininity in this way. It is also about having clean, shiny hair, teeth which are well cared for, good posture and taking pride in all aspects of your appearance.

Your body will be changing in all sorts of ways while you are pregnant. If your skin changes in texture, your normal foundation creams and powders may no longer suit you. You can experiment with new make-up techniques (see also page 28) or concentrate on enhancing a more natural look. Finding a 'look' that you like, such as using a minimum of make-up, will be useful in the early weeks after the baby is born, when feeding and caring for the baby and catching up with sleep seem to take most of your time. It isn't unusual to discover it's midday and you still have not dressed, let alone put on any make-up. You may also find that your skin reacts differently to the sun, in which case you will need to use a strong sun barrier.

During pregnancy the muscle shape of your legs may change and varicose veins may appear or become more pronounced. Wearing support tights, which are more comfortable in winter than summer, and putting your legs up as much as possible will ease any aching. Your breasts will not only grow larger – often to the delight of the flat chested – but the dark blue colour of the veins will also become more pronounced and your ribcage and hip bones will open out more during pregnancy. But nearly all these changes are temporary and after the birth your skin should soon return to normal and varicose veins will either disappear or become much less apparent. Three months or so after the birth your breasts will grow smaller again, your legs will slim down and your muscle tone improve. If you make time for doing exercises, particularly those which strengthen the muscles, and if you eat sensibly then there is no reason why you should not regain your figure, if not actually improve it!

Fluid retention in your hands may make it difficult to wear rings. If you do have a problem getting a ring off, hold your arm up above your head for a few minutes so that the fluid is able to drain downwards. Then, with a drop of washing-up liquid on the swollen finger and maybe a couple of ice cubes to help reduce any swelling, you should be able to remove the ring.

After the birth you may find your hands become dry and sore from being in water so much more, particularly if they come in contact with nappy sterilizing solution, which you may use to soak your baby's soiled clothes. You can protect your hands by wearing rubber gloves and using plenty of moisturizing hand cream.

'The daily changes to my shape I found amazing and somehow unbelievable. I kept wanting to touch my face and bump. Massaging my skin with a little oil not only satisfied this need but also refreshed my skin, making it feel silky and soft, which really helped me feel good.'

The way you look

Hair The hormone changes of pregnancy may mean either that your hair is thicker than normal, because fewer hairs are lost each day, or that it seems to fall out more easily. The latter often happens for about six months after the birth; in fact, hairs retained before the birth are being lost as well as your usual daily hair loss. Losing hair during pregnancy is quite normal and should not cause worry. Hair can also change to become either oilier or drier, glossier or duller.

Eyes Hormone changes may cause small alterations in the shape of the eye and can make wearing contact lenses uncomfortable. Extra fluid may also cause the skin below the eyes to become puffy.

Mouth Gums tend to bleed more easily (see page 26).

Skin Extra tiny blood vessels near the surface of the skin and an improved circulation add a natural blush to the skin. It may become oilier or drier than normal. Skin often darkens a little, particularly if you are dark haired or dark skinned, and you may have patches where the skin colour is uneven. Stretch marks may appear particularly on the hips, abdomen and breasts. These will fade to silvery lines after the birth.

Sweat Changes in the blood circulation cause you to feel hotter and you may also find you perspire more.

Breasts Changes in the breasts are one of the earliest signs of pregnancy. The glands enlarge, causing the breasts to become larger, firmer and more tender, and a tingling sensation is sometimes felt. From the middle of pregnancy drops of colostrum – the baby's first food if you breastfeed – may be secreted from the nipples and form tiny crusts which can be washed off. The skin around the nipple darkens and little raised sebaceous glands, which look like small bumps, appear; the nipple becomes softer. The breasts grow larger towards the end of the pregnancy and again in the early weeks of breastfeeding. They grow smaller when you have been breastfeeding for a couple of months or so.

Abdomen A line of brown pigment, the *linea nigra*, appears below your tummy button. More pronounced in dark-skinned women, it will fade after the birth.

Legs All the muscles strengthen and develop because of the weight that you will be putting on during your pregnancy.

Hands and feet The body gains 4.5 litres (14 pints) of fluid during pregnancy, sometimes even more. If this collects in the wrists, ankles, fingers and feet it is known as oedema. Oedema of the hands and feet is common and can be very uncomfortable. It is always checked at your antenatal visits.

Weight Fat is mainly put on over your trunk and thighs. See page 43.

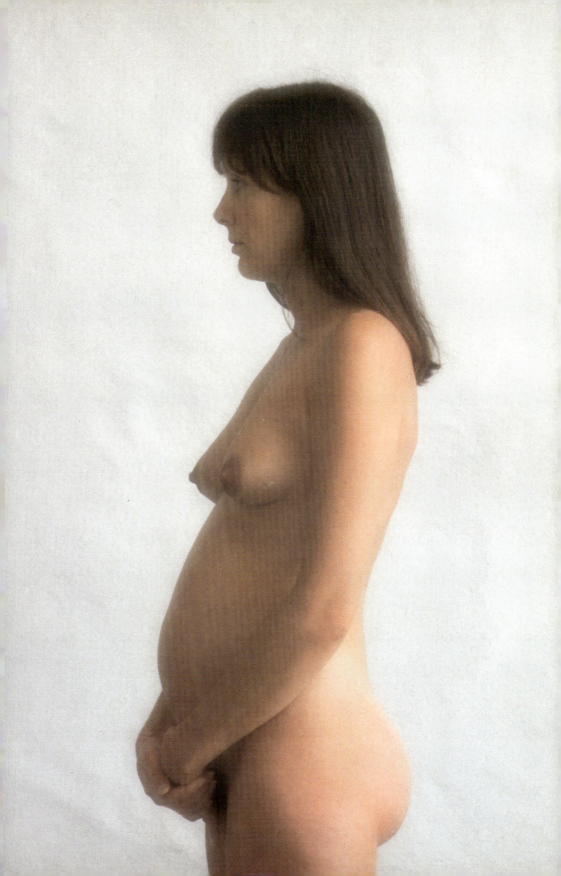

Keeping clean and fresh

A daily bath or shower is an important part of your beauty routine. The water should be warm rather than hot as hot water tends to dry the skin and, if your skin is itchy during pregnancy, high temperatures will make the problem worse. A small tub of bicarbonate of soda added to the bath can be soothing to itchy skin and it may be worth trying an unscented soap or a soapless cleansing bar if you find that your skin is very irritated.

Bathtime is a good opportunity to massage your tummy and you can also gently knead your nipples and stretch the areola or darker skin around them. A baby's suck is the most effective way of encouraging this but you can start by massaging and drawing out your nipples. Avoid using soap on them as it removes the natural oils which cleanse and lubricate them.

After your bath you may like to give yourself a massage with a little oil. If you have pronounced stretch marks you could massage oil around them. The aroma of a little eucalyptus or peppermint oil massaged on your throat and chest can ease your breathing if you are suffering from a stuffy nose, as sometimes occurs in pregnancy.

You may find that you are perspiring more towards the end of your pregnancy and this can be helped by using an antiperspirant to reduce the volume of sweat, instead of a simple deodorant. An increase in normal vaginal discharge is best coped with by using disposable pantie liners.

Caring for your teeth and gums
You should brush your teeth twice a day and use dental floss to clean between the teeth several times a week. Massaging your gums with a toothbrush twice a day will help to discourage infection and

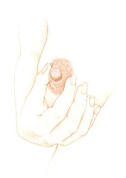

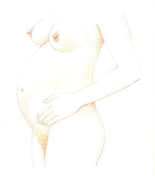

Gently kneading your nipples and stretching the areola around them makes them more supple and encourages the nipples to stick out for breastfeeding (left).

Massaging stretch marks stimulates the circulation which will help to nourish the skin (right).

inflammation. Pregnancy causes gums to become spongier and more prone to gingivitis – infection and bleeding around the gum margin. This can easily be controlled but if it is not the teeth may eventually loosen and the condition becomes irreversible.

Your dentist can help by giving your teeth a professional clean every few months; remember that dental treatment is free during pregnancy and for a year afterwards.

Your skin care

Oily skin needs particularly careful cleansing. You can use special lotions or simply rub a slice of cucumber over your face. If you don't wear make-up, then washing with soap and water is probably sufficient. You can test whether your skin is clean by wiping it with a little cleanser on cotton wool to see if any more dirt is removed.

Spots can be treated with a dab of witchhazel applied with a cotton bud or pad. Thorough cleansing with hypoallergenic products will also help. Do not be tempted to squeeze the spots as this could make the problem worse. Acne needs to be treated with an antibacterial wash or cleanser which can be prescribed by your doctor.

Dry skin needs plenty of moisturizing as well as thorough cleansing after using make-up. The most important effect of moisturizers on dry skin is to seal in the skin's natural lubricants. For this reason they are best avoided on oily skins.

Both oily and dry skin can benefit from a stimulating rub to remove the dead, surface cells and expose the fresh cells underneath. Known as exfoliation, this process helps dispel flaking, dry skin, unblocks pores and generally stimulates the circulation so nourishing the skin. If you use a flannel or a complexion brush, you can give your face a gentle scrub each day or you can use special cleansing grains or a mask every few days as recommended. The act of massaging in lotion is also both soothing and good for the skin.

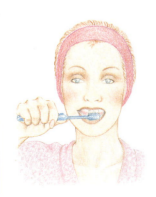

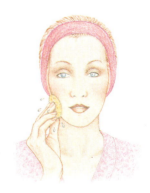

Gums tend to be spongier in pregnancy and you should brush them with a toothbrush when you clean your teeth (left).

Exfoliation – or giving your skin a stimulating rub with a flannel or buffing pad – helps remove flaking skin and unblock the pores (right).

Your make-up and hair

*H*ealthy skin is smooth, stretchy and supple. If you use make-up every day, your skin needs special care to keep it this way. Before putting on your make-up you should use a mild cleanser and then a toner or skin tonic to remove any remaining grease and to cool and prepare the skin so that make-up can be applied smoothly. Toners may contain herbal extracts or a spirit such as alcohol. If you have not used a heavy cleansing cream, you should need only a mild, herbal toner. Try to avoid spirit-based ones because they can have a hardening effect on the skin.

During pregnancy your skin can be particularly sensitive and it is best to use products which are described as hypoallergenic. This means that they are free from substances known to trigger off allergies. While you are pregnant, the colour and texture of your skin can change slightly and make-up can help with this. If you have any uneven patches of skin colour, for example, you can cover these up with foundation. The colour of your foundation should match your skin as closely as possible to avoid a contrast between the colour of your face and your neck. If your skin colour is heightened, you can use green cream or powder to tone down excessive redness. Dark shadows under the eyes can be lightened with highlighting cream or concealer but don't try too hard to disguise shadows or you may simply draw attention to them. You can use blusher to make your face look less round and a darker shade of foundation around the whole of the jaw line will also help.

If fluid retention is making your eyes puffy and your face fuller, soothe the eyes and reduce swelling by lying down for 10 minutes with some cotton-wool pads soaked in witchhazel or slices of cucumber placed on your eyelids. A lip salve will help retain

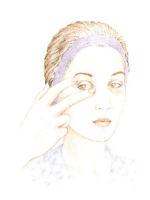

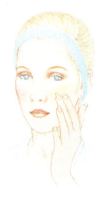

A little concealer can help to disguise any shadows under your eyes but apply it very lightly using a make-up brush or even just the tip of your finger (left).

If your complexion looks a little ruddy, you can tone it down with green cream or powder (right).

moisture if your lips become sore and dry. If you are very conscious of your fuller face, try wearing an eye-catching necklace to draw attention away from it. Other people, however, will probably not have noticed that your face is rounder. Facial roundness often makes the skin appear smoother. Add a pregnant bump and people usually think how young and well you look!

Easy hair care
Your hairdresser may be unwilling to give you any harsh hair treatments, such as perms or chemical dyes, while you are pregnant. This is partly a precaution to prevent strong chemicals from entering your blood stream through the hair roots and possibly getting through to the baby and partly because pregnancy can cause hair to behave in rather unpredictable ways.

If you wash your hair frequently, use a mild, frequent-wash shampoo as strong shampoos can irritate the scalp. Your hair will need frequent washing if it has become particularly oily, but avoid rubbing and brushing it too much as this will stimulate the sebaceous glands to produce more oil and it will soon look lank and lifeless again. If your hair is dry, it will help to use a conditioner when you wash it and a natural drying method.

If you need a hair cut in the early weeks after the baby is born, it is worth trying to find a hairdresser who will come to your home. Shop windows, local papers and your baby clinic are good places to look for advertisements. You will find that an easy hair style is particularly important after the baby is born. Newly washed hair is a tremendous morale booster and for many women their most important beauty aid. If your hair has to be carefully blow-dried or styled every time you wash it, you may be frustrated by your baby starting to cry before you have finished. Babies can wait while you rinse your hair but you will find it hard to ignore them for longer.

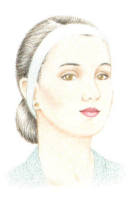

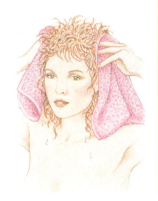

Blusher applied below the cheek bone and a darker foundation blended in around the jaw line can help to make your face look less round (left).

Try to find a hair style that can be towel dried and easily looked after to save you having to spend a lot of time on it (right).

Beauty sleep

Sleep disturbances are common during pregnancy and they can be worrying. If you are one of those people who is used to eight hours' uninterrupted sleep, you may feel quite unable to cope with less. Well-meaning remarks – like this being nature's way of preparing you for interrupted nights – are not only extremely unwelcome but probably untrue.

Sleep problems when you are pregnant are caused by a variety of reasons. You may have difficulty breathing easily in certain sleeping positions and anxiety or a general alertness can also make it difficult to relax. Worrying about not sleeping, however, is probably the best way of ensuring you don't sleep.

Bedtime routine

One of the most effective means of encouraging sleep is to develop a bedtime routine so that your mind 'learns' to wind down. Cleansing your face and giving it a gentle massage; a warm unhurried bath; a milky drink or a light snack such as a bowl of cereal; a warm or cool bed, depending on the time of year; and a few minutes' reading are often enough to cause sleepiness in many women. Once a routine is well established, then any part of it, such as the bath or the reading, may be sufficient. For the occasions when getting to sleep is particularly difficult, a massage (see page 98) or practising a relaxation technique (see page 93) may help.

Coping with sleeplessness

If you *are* waking in the night, then first of all you need to reassure yourself that it does not actually matter if you have less sleep than normal. Most people can adapt: we sleep most deeply in the first couple of hours after we fall asleep and that initial period is probably the most valuable – something that is worth remembering if you find yourself waking up in the small hours. Provided you lie quietly and are happy to let yourself daydream, you should soon go back to sleep. Even if you don't, your relaxation will have helped your body recover from the previous day. On the other hand, if you end up tossing and turning you will wear yourself out and probably wake up your partner. Sleeping in a different room from your partner may help: you can wriggle about as much as you like without the fear that you will be disturbing him.

If breathing is difficult or heartburn is a problem, you may find it much easier to sleep sitting up in an armchair with your feet raised and a quilt or sleeping bag round you. If you are longing to sleep face down but are prevented by your bump, then wrapping up warmly, sitting on an upright chair and resting with your head on your arms over a table may help. You will need to keep your feet warm so wear slippers with, perhaps, a hot-water bottle under your feet.

Getting up and going through the process of making yourself comfortable re-enacts the bedtime routine and this will often induce sleep. But if one night nothing seems to do the trick, it is better to spend the time doing something useful. Ironing or sewing in the middle of the night can be strangely soothing as well as giving you the satisfaction of a job done.

Your partner's needs

Having enough sleep after the baby is born is equally important for your partner if he is going to be able to help you and do more around the house in the early weeks. Accepting that one of you can sleep on the sofa rather than worrying that something may go wrong with your relationship if you don't stay in the same bed is often enough to ease an anxious situation. After a few weeks your baby should have developed a more predictable pattern of sleeping and feeding and your own sleep patterns will adjust so that you are much less tired.

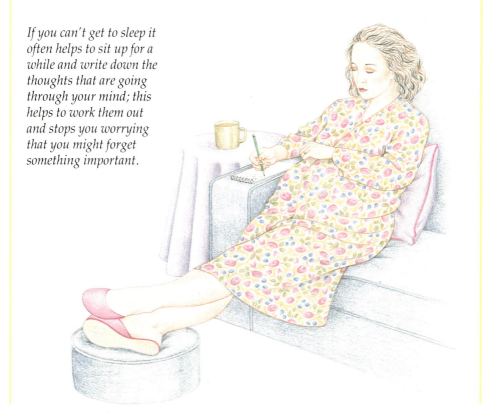

If you can't get to sleep it often helps to sit up for a while and write down the thoughts that are going through your mind; this helps to work them out and stops you worrying that you might forget something important.

After the baby is born

New babies have to be cared for round the clock. Of course they do sleep sometimes, but that's when you have to fit in everything else – eating, sleeping and keeping the household running. Until you get used to this, you may find yourself worrying that you are losing control of everything and becoming a bit of a frump. A simple programme for taking care of your appearance will be a great help.

A daily bath or shower is the first priority. It will keep you feeling fresh and also ensure that your breasts and vaginal area are kept clean. You also need to find a hairstyle that will require little more than a wash and rub or comb dry.

Structuring your day
In the early days you may find yourself anxious to establish a routine for your baby. Many new mothers feel that some predictable pattern will help to settle the baby and they can also feel very lost and vulnerable themselves, if they have only recently given up work, without some kind of schedule. Experienced mothers don't often have this problem because their other children usually have a well-established routine into which the baby soon fits. This does not mean that she has to wait to suit the convenience of the older children but she may, when necessary, be fed early and then given a few additional top-ups to keep her satisfied.

Creating some structure for your day or simply a check-list of things you expect to achieve is very important to your peace of mind at this time. And peace of mind will bring you that air of radiant motherhood that will enhance your natural looks.

If you aim, each day, to be dressed by a certain time, to get out and have some fresh air, to take some form of exercise, and to see or at least talk to a friend, you will be making a very good start. In the early days you may find this is as much as you can manage. But even if you can do no more, it really is worth starting off slowly rather than risking being disheartened if you have to slow down.

After about six weeks you will probably be feeling more settled as you and your hormones adjust after the birth and gradually you can take on more. However, it is worth remembering that it took nine months for your body to get ready for the birth. It will take several months before it readjusts.

*'Painting my nails was something thoroughly frivolous
which lifted my spirits and made me feel well-dressed, even
when I just had my dressing gown on!'*

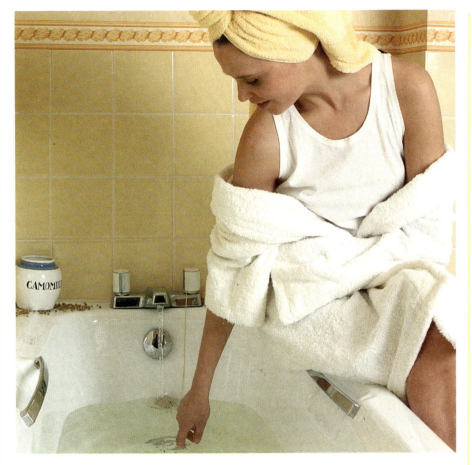

Your six-month beauty plan

Weeks 1 and 2 Make time for a daily bath or shower.

Weeks 3 and 4 Do some gentle exercises, have some fresh air and talk to at least one friend each day. Restart usual beauty and getting up routines.

Weeks 5 and 6 Make a hair appointment and maybe give yourself a facial. Join a postnatal exercise class, perhaps at a local health clinic or hospital.

Week 12 You can do much more vigorous exercise now. Your muscles are firmer though the ligaments are still soft. Your breasts will be smaller even though, if you are breastfeeding, you are producing more milk.

6 months Talk to your doctor or health visitor about going on a slimming diet if you need to, once weaning is established. Any extra hair loss should have stopped. You should be feeling fit and clear-headed enough to go back to work or to start adult education classes but you may still feel tired if the baby is waking up at night.

YOUR PREGNANCY
≈ *WARDROBE* ≈

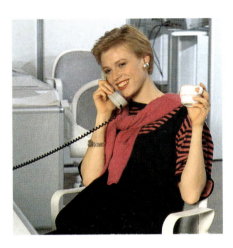

*Y*ou don't become a totally different person when you are pregnant so why change the style of clothes you wear? If you keep to the sort of clothes you normally wear, with adaptations to accommodate your changing shape, you will feel comfortable and your pregnancy will seem a more natural part of your life.

Start to plan your wardrobe by looking through as many magazines and catalogues as possible to get some idea of what might suit you. You don't have to look just at maternity wear; loose ordinary clothes may be equally suitable.

Dungarees and jumpsuits have to be long in the crutch and generous at the thigh and not just baggy around the middle to accommodate your growing bump. Tops and jackets have to be roomy round the front *and* the back as your bust grows and your ribcage expands in the latter half of pregnancy. Wrap your arms round yourself when you try tops on. If the garment feels tight, reject it. If you buy clothes before you get larger, take a small cushion with you when you try them on to check that the hemline will not ride up too much at the front compared with the back.

Construct your wardrobe of interchangeable clothes so that you can vary your 'look' without buying vast numbers of garments. A few basics will go a long way if you choose them cleverly.

One of the awkward times to deal with is the in-between stage when your old clothes are uncomfortable but you are swamped by maternity wear. For some women this happens at around four months, as waist-fitting clothes become difficult to do up. Others start growing out of their clothes earlier than this and yet others don't noticeably expand until six months. A lot depends on how fitted your ordinary clothes are. If you favour styles that are loose and roomy, they'll go on fitting you well into your pregnancy. This in-between time is common for a few weeks during pregnancy and for several months after the birth.

The most comfortable clothes for both in-between stages are separates: skirts and trousers with elasticated waists, soft track suits, harem trousers, sweat shirts, T-shirts and fisherman's smocks. For pregnancy, loose dresses which can be gathered with a belt are useful but after the birth dresses can be inconvenient. They are awkward for breastfeeding and the whole outfit has to be changed if your baby is sick over you.

Clothes that can be layered are useful for changes in the weather as well as in your own body temperature. Natural fibres may also be more comfortable than synthetics, particularly in summer.

Accessories can transform an outfit so that casual clothes can double up for more formal wear if you add a smart jacket or blouse, jewellery or a scarf. If you are looking for clothes which will also be suitable after the baby is born, they must be easily washable. Clothes which need careful laundering or dry cleaning are impractical. Babies don't just make their own clothes messy; they can dirty yours almost as quickly. Clothes that are comfortable and convenient for breast-feeding are also worth considering if you are planning to feed the baby yourself. Two-piece outfits that can be pulled up from the waist are very practical. However, don't forget that time passes and clothes which are suitable for pregnancy may not be appropriate six months later when the season has changed!

'Wearing comfortable sporty clothes helped me feel healthy, which I think actually made me take more care of what I ate and encouraged me to exercise more.'

Casual clothes

When you want to relax yet still look good, choose coordinated clothes that fit well to help you feel your best. Tops or skirts that are too short or too tight will accentuate your bump rather than enhance your figure, and simply contrive to make you feel awkward and uncomfortable.

A pair of maternity denim or cord jeans are a versatile basis for your casual wardrobe. These can look good with a polo-neck top,

A pinafore dress is an ideal casual style that can be varied to suit many occasions by changing the shirt you wear underneath. The same tops can be worn with maternity trousers provided they are long enough to cover your bump. Maternity trousers have an elasticated waist or an adjustable fastening so that they expand with you.

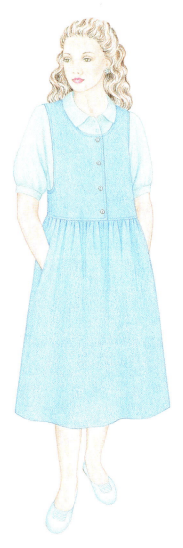

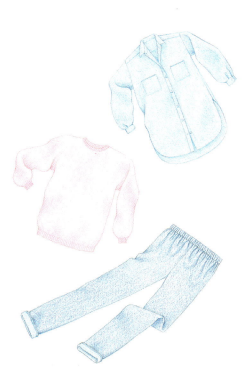

sweat shirt or T-shirt. A maternity denim pinafore dress is also a good neutral accompaniment for different coloured tops. Denim or cord are comfortable during most months of the year, and by adding or removing layers you can adapt to almost any weather.

Casual shoes should be low-heeled and comfortable. Trainers or canvas shoes are ideal, especially as lace-ups can 'give' if your feet are slightly swollen or enlarged because of looser ligaments. High boots may become uncomfortable later in pregnancy because your leg muscles may be larger from carrying your extra weight. They should return to their former size after the birth.

Cord trousers are stylish, comfortable and can be mixed and matched with a variety of tops. A long polo-neck looks casual yet neat whereas a baggy T-shirt is fun and practical, especially teamed with a large shirt or jacket. In colder weather a bright scarf will both warm and cheer you.

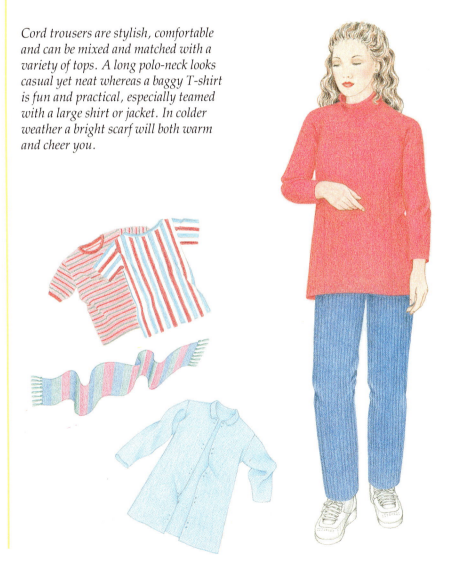

Formal wear

Special occasions warrant special clothes for you to feel your best. Although you're pregnant you will still want to be appropriately dressed. If you have difficulty finding something you like in maternity wear, you can try a loose-fitting style that is not specifically designed for a mother-to-be. Alternatively, a really stunning jacket which will also suit you after the birth can be added to a basic black skirt and smart blouse for a dressy evening out.

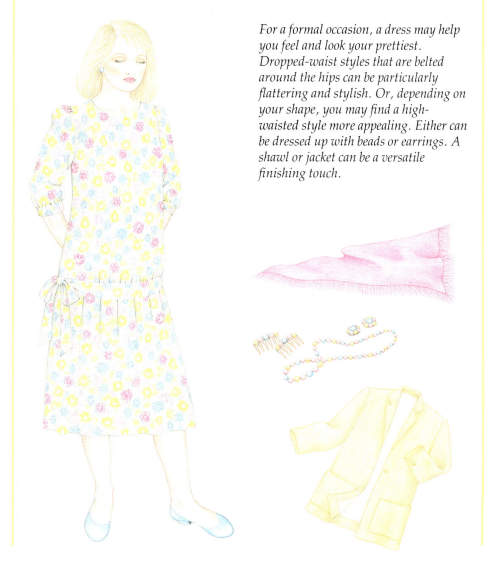

For a formal occasion, a dress may help you feel and look your prettiest. Dropped-waist styles that are belted around the hips can be particularly flattering and stylish. Or, depending on your shape, you may find a high-waisted style more appealing. Either can be dressed up with beads or earrings. A shawl or jacket can be a versatile finishing touch.

Wear smart, low-heeled shoes to complement your outfit. High heels may make you shift your weight forward, causing backache and tired feet and legs. In flat shoes you will find it easier to stand well with your back straight, without pushing your bump forward.

Looking smart for work may require new outfits but again the secret is to mix and match with interchangeable tops and skirts. When buying skirts, those that are fairly full are often more flattering towards the end of pregnancy when you may want to sit with your legs apart or to raise them on a stool. Knowing you can sit comfortably will make you feel more confident.

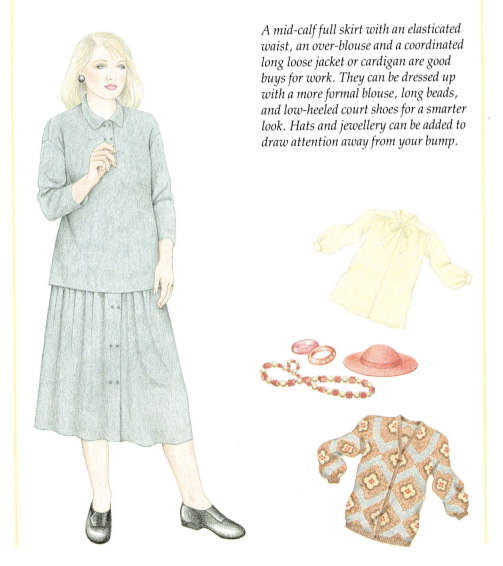

A mid-calf full skirt with an elasticated waist, an over-blouse and a coordinated long loose jacket or cardigan are good buys for work. They can be dressed up with a more formal blouse, long beads, and low-heeled court shoes for a smarter look. Hats and jewellery can be added to draw attention away from your bump.

Nightwear and underwear

*B*y about the tenth week of pregnancy your breasts will have enlarged considerably. Since breast tissue contains no muscle, you will need a bra that supports comfortably and firmly. Unless it is very adjustable, you may need to buy several bras at different stages of your pregnancy to accommodate your larger ribcage as well. To determine the size you will need, measure across the fullest part of your breast and under your breast. The difference between the two measurements will indicate the cup size required and the smaller measurement the bra size. Wide, adjustable straps are most comfortable and give the best support.

If you are planning to breastfeed, you can buy a nursing bra when you are about seven or eight months pregnant. Do make sure that there is room for expansion. Nursing bras should open at the front or have drop cups to allow the baby easy access to the breast. Bras with elasticated fabric over the breasts should be avoided because the elastic can constrict and block the milk ducts and this can cause your breasts to become very painful.

Pants, girdles and tights

Bikini-style pants can be worn throughout pregnancy, but make sure they are cotton to help relieve any thrush. After the birth, you may want some stretchy fabric ones to support tender tummy muscles and hold a sanitary towel securely. If your ligaments are painful during pregnancy, you may find a maternity girdle helpful.

Dark coloured tights help to make your legs look slimmer, while patterned or brightly coloured tights can liven up a neutral skirt or

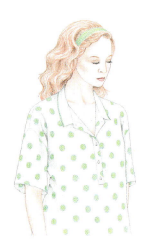

Cotton nightdresses are comfortable if you find you get warm at night. Sleep bras give relief if your breasts sometimes feel heavy (left).

A good bra provides support and fits well over your shoulders and around your back and ribcage. If possible, try several on to find the one that's best for you (right).

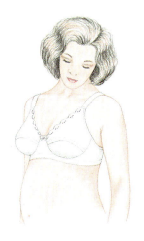

dress. Maternity tights are available or you can wear extra-large tights back to front. Support tights or stockings can be extremely comfortable and they conceal as well as relieve varicose veins. They are now available in a variety of attractive styles.

Your hospital case

If you ask at the antenatal clinic, you may find that you can choose what you are going to wear during labour. Hospital gowns are usually unattractive and can inhibit movement. You may feel happier and more confident in a T-shirt and a pair of pants (until your waters have broken), a comfortable nightshirt or a loose-fitting, sleeveless dress; the important point is that whatever you choose should be clean, washable and not cumbersome. You will need enough nightdresses, nightshirts or T-shirts to have a change every day and maybe even more frequently if your baby has accidents on you. Whatever you choose to wear, it should open down the front to the waist or be easy to pull up if you are breastfeeding. You don't have to wear nightclothes during the daytime in hospital. Wearing day clothes such as a lightweight tracksuit can help you feel more in control and ready to cope. You will be expected to care for yourself and your baby from the very beginning and that can be difficult to do in hospital, lying in bed in a nightie.

One of the most important items in your hospital case should be an attractive dressing gown. You want to make sure you like yourself in those first photographs with the baby. And later on at home, you may find yourself regularly opening the door to midwives and other visitors in your dressing gown. It has to be comfortable and roomy enough to cover your bust, which will enlarge considerably three or four days after the birth whether you breastfeed or not.

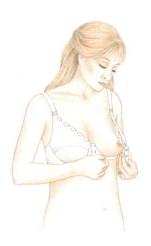

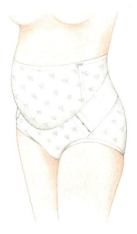

A front-opening bra for breastfeeding gives the baby easy access to the breast and provides individual support for your breasts (left).

An adjustable maternity girdle can supply added support for your back and abdomen when the pregnancy hormones cause your ligaments to stretch (right).

41

≈ *YOUR DIET* ≈

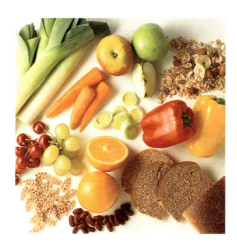

*O*bviously, your body changes both inside and out as pregnancy progresses. A fetus can only grow if it gets sufficient nutrients and it takes its supplies, via the placenta, from your body stores. But your metabolism is changing subtly to cope with these demands. Although the body needs roughly an extra 200 kilocalories a day, double the normal amount of calcium and vitamin C and a third more iron during pregnancy, a healthy woman eating a balanced diet with plenty of fresh foods has to make few, if any, changes to what she eats. Instead, her body adapts by wasting fewer nutrients from the food she eats and becoming much more efficient about what it does use. For example, the baby needs most calcium in the last three months of pregnancy when he is growing rapidly, but the mother's body begins saving it from the very beginning.

Just how smoothly the body adapts to pregnancy – even if you are feeling sick, tired and thoroughly miserable – has yet to be fully appreciated. But, although nature may be highly efficient, she is not foolproof – particularly when it comes to coping with the effects of drugs and diseases. Uncertainty still exists about which substances cross the placenta and can affect your unborn baby. (See page 45 for more information about alcohol, caffeine and other stimulants.) Most medication is best avoided in pregnancy. If you are in *any* doubt about the safety of a medication you are taking, then check with your doctor or chemist, making sure that they know you are pregnant. You should also check if you are breastfeeding.

Gaining weight
You will probably find yourself gaining weight when the baby inside you is only just bigger than your thumbnail, about eight weeks into pregnancy. Weight gain commonly ranges anywhere from 6.3 to 19kg (14–42lb). Some women will gain nothing whereas others put on even more without any ill-effects to themselves or the baby. The baby does not account for the entire weight increase; at birth that can be broken down as follows: the baby itself weighs about 3.3kg (7¼lb), the placenta 0.6kg (1¼lb), the uterus 0.9kg (2lb), extra breast tissue 0.4kg (½lb), extra blood 1.2kg (2½lb), extra fat 3.5kg (7¾lb) and extra fluid 2.6kg (5¾lb).

How much weight you gain is not something over which you have much control. Your body is very good at guarding against weight loss. What you can influence is *what* you give your body to store. What you eat during pregnancy is important for your fitness and health and for ensuring that your body has plentiful supplies of minerals and certain vitamins if you plan to breastfeed. To ensure your own good health and that of your baby, make sure that your diet is balanced and contains the nutrients your body needs. Pregnancy is an ideal time to establish healthy eating habits. If your diet consists of too many sugary and fatty foods, now is the time to start enjoying fresh fruit and vegetables, wholemeal bread and other unprocessed grains and pulses.

Your doctor and midwife are likely to be much more interested in the rate at which you gain weight rather than the actual amount you put on. Any sudden losses or gains or a failure to put on any weight at all need to be checked.

Just as important as thinking about what you should eat to protect the baby inside you is to think about what sort of diet your baby will have after birth. It is important to realize that a child does not simply grow in size after birth, but that its internal organs continue to develop. A healthy diet during a child's growing years lays the foundation for health and fitness in later life.

Eating for health

*A*djusting to healthy eating takes time, and pregnancy is an excellent opportunity to begin to put the principles into practice. You should soon begin to feel better for it and this is the best incentive to give your body any extra nutrients you may need.

A healthy diet contains plenty of fruits, vegetables and cereal foods (like pasta, rice, bread and potatoes); moderate amounts of lean meats, fish, poultry, dairy foods, eggs, nuts and beans; and only small amounts of fats, oils and sugar. Follow these recommendations and you will be absorbing ample amounts of vitamins and minerals, plenty of protein, adequate fibre and enough fat and sugar. It means choosing dishes in which the main ingredient is a carbohydrate-rich food like rice or pasta, with a sauce containing some meat, poultry, fish or beans and plenty of vegetables, served with extra vegetables or a side salad and a basket of bread, and fresh fruit to follow.

This sort of meal is typical of much traditional Mediterranean and Eastern cuisine and many people eat like this occasionally. You simply have to do so more often. Eating in this way helps you use more fibre-rich foods and fewer of the less healthy fatty foods. Provided you keep a check on these two components, the rest of your healthy eating regime should take care of itself.

Vitamin and mineral supplements

A normally healthy woman should not need to supplement her diet with extra vitamins and minerals during pregnancy. However, there are some medical conditions for which supplements may be pre-scribed as a safety measure or as part of treatment.

Iron tablets used to be given to all pregnant women. It is now known that it is normal for the quantity of haemoglobin in a pregnant woman's blood to fall below the normal 12–13 grams per 100 millimetres of blood. Only when the level falls to 10½ grams or below or when examination of the blood cells under a microscope shows that their shape is no longer normal are tablets prescribed. Foods like red meat, beans, citrus fruits, fresh green vegetables and wholemeal bread should help keep your blood healthy.

Asian women and their babies are particularly susceptible to vitamin D deficiency. Vitamin D is needed to lay down calcium in bones and a deficiency commonly causes rickets. Asian women may therefore be prescribed a vitamin D and calcium supplement as a precaution. Vitamin D is found in few foods. The best source is sunlight on the skin and the most useful food sources are fortified margarine, fatty fish like herring, kippers and salmon, eggs and fortified breakfast cereals. A vitamin supplement is sometimes

This appetizing and easily prepared meal of fibre-rich foods is high in vitamins and minerals and low both in fats and added sugar.

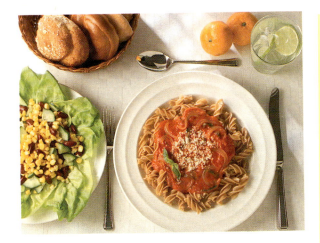

prescribed before pregnancy for women who are at risk of having a baby with spina bifida. There is some evidence that such women may be either deficient in certain B vitamins, like folic acid, or that enough of the vitamins they get from food are not passed on to the fetus. Vitamin supplements should really only be taken if prescribed by a doctor because it is possible to overdose. However, if you have been giving yourself a general vitamin supplement in no more than the medically recommended amounts, you are unlikely to have done yourself or your baby any harm.

Alcohol, caffeine and herbal remedies

Alcohol, coffee, tea and many herbal remedies all contain pharmacologically active agents. This means that when you consume a large amount of any of them they can act like a drug. Finding out what size of dose is harmful to you is extremely difficult so the only safe course is to avoid them. However, this is not only harsh, and in some cases impractical, advice but it can also cause great concern if you regularly took any of them before you knew you were pregnant.

At the moment the consensus of expert opinion is that alcohol should be avoided, though an occasional glass or two of wine is unlikely to be harmful. In the USA doctors recommend that caffeine intake should be no more than that from six cups of coffee or 14 cups of tea or cola drinks a day. If you drink a lot of coffee, then it is worth changing over to a decaffeinated type.

Herbal remedies have only recently begun to be studied by the medical profession. But there is a growing body of trained medical herbalists and their advice is that people should not treat themselves as herbal treatments, used wrongly, may be useless or highly poisonous. Contact the National Institute of Medical Herbalists (see page 125) for a list of registered members.

The value of fibre

There's more to increasing the fibre in your diet than simply eating wholemeal, instead of white, bread or an extra piece of fruit each day. Both measures will certainly take you in the right direction but, unless you already eat a lot of bread, fruit and vegetables, they will not be enough to achieve the recommended 30 grams of fibre a day, which is half as much again as most people eat.

A few guidelines are all you need. Listed below are small, average and large servings of food which contain about 3 grams of fibre each. Salad vegetables, such as lettuce and cucumber, have not been included: they contain only tiny quantities of fibre. You need to eat 10 of these servings a day to get the recommended daily intake. For example, one bowl of high-fibre cereal, one slice of wholemeal toast, one round of wholemeal bread sandwiches, three portions of vegetables, one portion of beans or nuts (maybe added to a meat dish), an orange and a banana would add up to 30 grams of fibre and give you plenty of vitamins and minerals. (As beans are a common cause of wind, dried beans must be properly soaked and cooked, otherwise buy canned beans.)

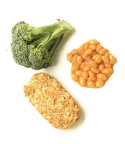 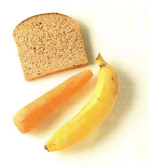 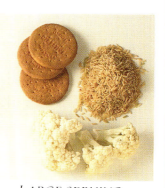

SMALL SERVING
Broad beans, butter beans, broccoli, leeks, peas, plantain, spinach, sweetcorn, yam, lentils, 2 tbsp baked beans, blackberries, dried apricots, raspberries, dried prunes, All Bran, 1 Shredded Wheat or Weetabix, 1 slice wholemeal bread

AVERAGE SERVING
French beans, runner beans, sprouts, cabbage, carrots, swede, sweet potato, chips, stewed plums, gooseberries, medium banana, 2 small apples, 2 tangerines, handful of dried fruit or nuts, Puffed Wheat, 2 crispbreads, 1 slice of fruitcake

LARGE SERVING
Aubergine, cauliflower, turnip, new potatoes in their skins, red kidney beans, parsnips, strawberries, 1 large orange, 1 grapefruit, 2 pears, nectarines or peaches, muesli, brown rice, wholemeal pasta or 3 digestive biscuits

Playing down fatty foods

It isn't always easy to keep track of the fats in our food but it is important to do so for your general health and because fatty foods seem to be responsible for some problems in pregnancy, such as nausea (see following page). Of course, they are present in the obviously fatty foods like butter, margarine, oil, cooking fats and cream, but they are also often 'hidden' in foods, most notably in fresh meat (in the lean as well as the fat), meat products (like meat pies and sausages), milk, eggs, cheese, biscuits, salad dressings, mayonnaise, ice-cream, chips, crisps, cakes and all manner of pastries.

The average woman eats about 90 grams of fat a day whereas the recommended maximum is 80 grams and a little less is even better. Now that more low-fat foods are appearing on the market it is easier to find alternatives to your favourite foods. Listed below are the most important changes you can make to your diet.

Milk Use semi-skimmed or skimmed milk instead of silver-top. If you drink half a pint a day, changing to skimmed milk could lose that excess 10 grams; semi-skimmed milk would leave you with 5 grams still to shed. If you are also increasing your fibre-rich foods, you may need to cut down a little more to lose the extra fat you may be spreading on bread, if you are now eating more sandwiches.

Ice-cream and cream Use low-fat yoghurt instead.

Cheese Check the fat content on the label. Choose edam, cottage cheese or the low-fat versions of hard cheeses instead of cheeses like cheddar and cream cheese.

Cooking fats, oils, butter and margarine Make sure your cooking fats, salad oils or margarines and spreads are labelled 'high in polyunsaturates'. These fats are just as fatty and rich in calories but the fat is of a healthier type. Beware of the term 'vegetable fat' on labels; it is no guarantee that the fats are healthier. Oils to choose are corn, soya, sunflower, safflower and grapeseed.

Meat Eat meat only once a day and eat more chicken and turkey. Make sure red meat is lean, and when preparing stews, casseroles or mince dishes, replace half the meat with pulses and root vegetables. Fish, as long as it isn't fried, is an excellent low-fat alternative.

Salad dressings Go for low-fat or non-oily varieties. You can simply use lemon juice, a mixture of vinegar and stock or fruit juice, or low-fat yoghurt flavoured with fresh chives or mint.

Potatoes Choose baked potatoes instead of chips, though thick-cut oven chips are not too fatty.

Bread A basket of fresh bread on the table at mealtimes is one way to eat bread without adding butter or margarine.

Cakes and biscuits If you must have them, choose plain or fruit varieties and those made with wholemeal flour or oatmeal.

Food problems in pregnancy

There are a number of common problems in pregnancy that are associated in some way with food and the digestive system. A simple change of diet or routine can often alleviate the problem.

Nausea

Feeling sick and retching is much more common than actually being sick during pregnancy. Unless you are vomiting frequently, you will not jeopardize your baby's health. Although it is commonest in the earliest weeks, some women do suffer with sickness for longer. Nobody really knows what the reason is, although urinary-tract infections can cause nausea. Nor is it a simple problem to treat as there appears to be no single remedy. Most of all, you need understanding and support from other people.

Nausea is often aggravated by food and drink, hunger, tiredness, strong smells, unpleasant sights, travel, worry and getting up in a hurry. The foods and drinks which seem the most likely irritants are tea, coffee, fatty food, milk, yoghurt, cheese, meat and chicken, spicy foods, wine, fruit juice and squash. Those which can be best tolerated are often items which the sufferer does not normally eat.

Foods which may be better tolerated are bland or salty or herb-flavoured foods, such as bread, potatoes, rice, pasta, cottage cheese, savoury biscuits, crisps, drinks made with yeast or beef extract, herb teas, fizzy drinks like soda water, mint sweets and fresh fruit. When you do find something that doesn't upset you, eat it slowly in small quantities rather than in one large meal. There may be one food, like an apple, which can be easily carried around with you for emergencies to help you stop an attack of nausea. When you feel sick, do everything slowly and practise deep breathing until the sick feeling has passed to release any muscle tension (see page 94).

Indigestion

Indigestion is caused partly by the growing uterus pressing on the stomach and partly because the softening of muscles at the base of the oesophagus, the tube between mouth and stomach, encourages the regurgitation of small quantities of food and stomach acid, resulting in the sensation known as 'heartburn'.

You can help prevent indigestion by sitting as straight as possible at mealtimes, eating little and often, chewing your food thoroughly and eating when you feel relaxed rather than tense. It takes longer for food to leave the stomach during pregnancy so after meals it is better to keep upright. Walking about is often more comfortable than reclining with your feet up. If heartburn at night is your problem, you

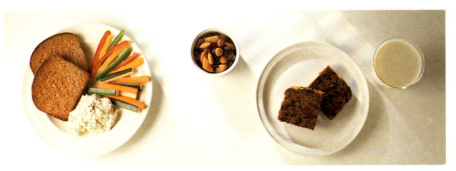

Some healthy snacks (see page 51) that may help if you can't cope with large meals or are extra hungry in pregnancy.

need to sleep well propped up, and it may help if you have your main meal in the middle of the day. You can also ask your doctor or pharmacist for a calcium or magnesium-based antacid.

Constipation

The intestines can become sluggish during pregnancy as they relax following the hormone changes the body undergoes. Iron tablets can also cause constipation: it may be worth asking your doctor or midwife if you can change brands or stop taking them. The best foods for relieving constipation are those which contain cereal fibre, such as wholemeal bread and high-bran breakfast cereals; prunes are helpful too. If you can increase your fibre intake to 30 grams a day and drink plenty of water, constipation shouldn't be a problem. Exercise will also help maintain the muscle tone of your internal organs. When you go to the lavatory, you may find it helps to sit well back on the seat with your feet supported in a squatting position.

Constipation is a common problem in the early days after the birth and it is often aggravated by low-fibre hospital food. Taking in your own high-bran cereal and dried prunes is a good idea. If you have stitches, it will help if you support them with a wadge of tissue on the perineum when you try to open your bowels.

Food poisoning

Particular care needs to be taken about food hygiene in pregnancy as food poisoning can have very serious effects on the fetus and the newborn baby. Thoroughly wash salad, fruit and vegetables; keep cooked foods well separated from raw foods and whenever possible store food in the fridge. When you reheat foods, make sure they are piping hot. Whenever possible avoid buying chilled ready-to-eat foods, soft ripened cheeses like brie, camembert or the blue-veined varieties, and ready-prepared salads.

After the baby is born

You may not look that much smaller immediately after your baby is born but over the next few days you will lose most of the extra fluid put on in pregnancy, and during the following weeks your stomach will flatten and tighten up as it regains its muscle tone.

Only about a quarter of the average weight gain in pregnancy is extra fat. This body fat is the storehouse for the extra calories needed for breastfeeding. So, if you breastfeed, in theory you should not need to eat very much more than normal to give your baby all the nutrients needed for growth and you should slowly shed that extra weight through the first six months after the birth. However, many women find they do not lose this extra half stone until they have finally weaned the baby.

Breastfeeding and appetite

Your appetite may be much greater while you are breastfeeding and, indeed, you may find that in the early months the start of a breastfeed triggers off hunger pangs and a sudden thirst. Whether you feel hungry or not, you should eat well. Your body may not use its fat stores any quicker if you eat less and may even cut down the milk supply so that your baby grows more slowly.

Eating in the early months

Whether you breastfeed or not, you will need to eat properly if you are to cope with the demands of a small baby. But eating properly does not have to mean three cooked meals a day. You probably will not have the time or the inclination for more than one main meal.

In the early months after the birth you may feel you want to indulge in chocolate biscuits and sweets. These can be soothing, but you do risk establishing habits which will be difficult to break. A much better idea is to have snack meals made from healthy foods.

Below are some ideas for healthy filling snacks which are quick and easy to prepare. Whatever snack you devise, if you make sure it has some bread or cereal-based food, some fresh fruit, salad or vegetable, and some cheese, meat, milk, beans or equivalent protein you will have a basic nutritional balance. And if the foods from the first two groups form the greater part of the snack it is likely to be all the healthier. None of these snacks is a substitute for a meal but six or seven in addition to one good-sized meal supplying approximately 600–900 kilocalories will give you the daily 2750 kilocalories you need while breastfeeding. If you are bottlefeeding, four or five of these snacks in addition to a meal of about 600 calories will add up to the average woman's daily requirement of 2150 kilocalories.

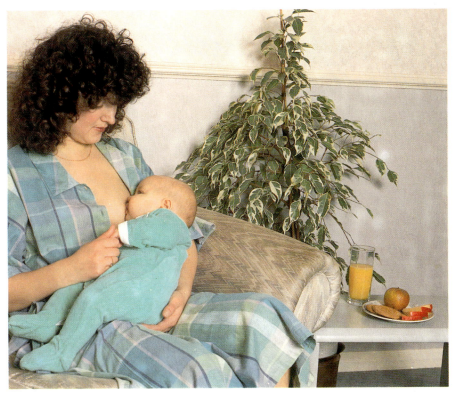

Snack-meal suggestions

☐ 2 Weetabix with semi-skimmed milk, sweetened with chopped fruit   *270 kcals*

☐ 3 digestive biscuits, 37g (1½oz) edam-type cheese and a glass of fruit juice   *400 kcals*

☐ 1 round of wholemeal sandwiches, spread with polyunsaturated margarine, and chicken and tomato filling   *260 kcals*

☐ 1 slice of fruitcake and glass of semi-skimmed milk   *360 kcals*

☐ 2 slices of wholemeal toast, smoked mackerel pâté, lettuce and red pepper   *350 kcals*

☐ 2 tbsp mixed beans, 2 tbsp sweetcorn and 2 tbsp chopped cucumber, tomato or other salad vegetable or fruit, with 1 tbsp french dressing   *230 kcals*

☐ Beans on wholemeal toast, spread with polyunsaturated margarine, 1 poached egg and a piece of fruit   *320 kcals*

☐ 2 handfuls (50g/2oz) of nuts and raisins   *220 kcals*

☐ 1 apple/pear (60 kcals), 1 banana (80 kcals), 1 orange (40 kcals), 1 peach/melon wedge (50 kcals) and 1 brown bread roll (155 kcals)

≈ *YOUR JOB* ≈

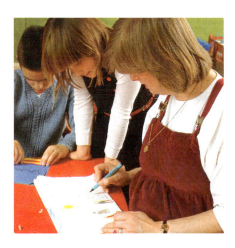

*I*t is usually best to tell your employers as soon as you know you are pregnant. Letting them know early on gives you time to sound out how they react and how supportive they are likely to be when you have to decide at what point before the birth to stop working and whether you will return to work afterwards. It also gives them time to plan how they can cover your job while you are away and enables them to make allowances if you suffer from sickness or extreme tiredness in the early months.

Knowing your rights

There are laws which entitle you to certain basic rights, such as free dental treatment, a maternity grant and maternity leave with protection for your job, depending on how long you have worked for your present employer and the number of hours per week you work. Some large companies provide additional benefits. Ask the personnel department for details of these and your state benefits. You can also discuss with them the possibility of returning to work and whether your job will be held open for you. The personnel department or your trade union should also be able to tell you of your company's safety procedures. This is particularly important if you have to work with dangerous chemicals, radiographic equipment, farm animals or factory machinery. If you have to do a lot of physical work which involves lifting heavy weights, other work may be found for you.

Visual display units such as those accompanying computers and word processors are not believed to present any health risks to pregnant women according to the National Radiological Protection Board, although this is still under investigation as a precaution. But if you are worried or find the atmosphere stressful, your employer may be able to find other work for you.

Every woman is entitled to paid time off for antenatal clinic appointments but not every employer will do the same for antenatal classes. This is something worth negotiating, especially if you stay on at work beyond the twenty-ninth week.

Programming your working day
Although many women can 'forget' they are pregnant during the hours of work, some are so tired or keen to start preparations for the baby that pregnancy and work create conflicting demands. For example, if a rest in the middle of the day would really help or you want to do exercises during the day because you are too tired in the evenings, then this should be discussed at work. Few employers would object to you resting during your lunch hour and increasingly people are arriving at the office early to exercise at a gym.

When to stop working
When you give up work before the birth is a very personal decision. Complications such as high blood pressure may force you to leave work before you intended. But you may be able to work right up to the end of pregnancy if you are healthy and want to carry on.

Most women prefer to stop working when they are between 28 and 34 weeks pregnant to gain their full maternity benefits and maximum time off work. Having these weeks off before the birth can be an opportunity for getting used to being at home during the day.

'I often need to put my legs up during meetings. I find that if I simply tell them I am going to do this, without making a fuss or apologizing for it, they just accept it.'

Going back to work

W hatever your intention about returning to work while you are pregnant, you may change your mind after the baby is born. You may find that being at home with your baby is fulfilling, challenging and the most rewarding experience of your life. Or you may decide that you need the stimulation of work and the company of other adults to keep your mind active. Alternatively, if you need the money, going back to work may be something you seem to have little choice about. Whatever decision you make, be confident in it. In most women's experience it is probably easier to plan to go back to work and then not go because you have changed your mind than to plan to stay at home, give in your notice and then find you want to return to work after all.

Time to take stock
In theory, there are at least four alternatives open to you when you take time off to have a baby. In practice, not all these possibilities may be available, particularly if you are in an area where there are few job opportunities or adult education facilities.

Going back to the same job This is probably the most straightforward choice, provided you can get adequate childcare. The law protects your rights to go back to work full-time, provided you have worked for your employer for a statutory (legally required) length of time and for a certain number of hours per week.
Finding a different job This is also reasonably straightforward, if you are prepared to take a job for which you are over-qualified. Again, you'll have to explore the childcare possibilities.
Training for a new job Learning a new skill or acquiring additional qualifications can be a worthwhile venture. Many further education colleges operate a crèche, solving the problem of finding a childminder. A course will provide mental stimulus, and may make you more employable if and when you do want to go back to work.

Acquiring extra skills does not necessarily imply academic study. You can also get involved in voluntary work, which can teach you organizational skills and may bring out unknown talents.
Working part-time You and your partner could share childminding responsibilities if you can both make flexible work arrangements. But hardest of all is the task of finding a part-time job with status equivalent to that of a previous full-time job. A few employers are exploring the potential of long-term career breaks, job-sharing and other forms of part-time employment, but most are still resistant to such changes. Those organizations which have tried to be more

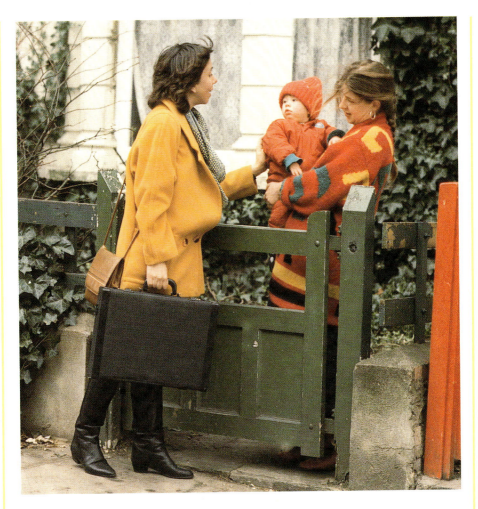

flexible have found a number of advantages. Job-sharing enables them to keep valued members of staff, costs are reduced because there is generally less absenteeism (staff use their own time for medical appointments and illness) and more work gets done.

If part-time work seems to be the solution for you, you must prepare your case carefully. Assess the likely administrative problems and find examples of workplaces where a similar scheme has been tried out successfully. Identify the advantages as well as the pitfalls (with solutions, of course). The better your homework, the greater your chance of creating the job or career break you want.

For more information contact New Ways to Work. This London-based organization issues leaflets and a newsletter which could be useful elsewhere. Another contact is the Working Mothers Association. For addresses see page 125.

Childcare choices

*F*inding reliable help can make or break a smooth return to work. You need to find someone you can trust and at a cost you can afford. In this country, two thirds of working women with very young children have a relative, or partner, who is able to look after the child; the remaining third use childminders, nannies, and day nurseries or crèches. If you do not have a partner or member of the family you can call on, you will have to consider one of the other options. What is available to you will depend much on your family circumstances, where you live and the age of your child.

If you intend to return to work by the time the baby is three months old, you should look into all possibilities before the baby arrives. Your health visitor may be able to advise you on the facilities in your area. Otherwise, you need to start looking for a childminder two to three months before you plan to return to work so that you and your baby have a couple of weeks to try out the arrangements. Childminders and day nurseries have waiting lists and nannies need time to work out their notice.

Childminders
The advantages of a childminder are that she probably lives locally, can provide continuity of care and is experienced, and there will usually be other children around. Your local authority has a list of registered childminders. Officially she should have only one baby under 12 months and no more than three children under five, including her own.

Registration is no guarantee of quality and it is wise to make a few discreet enquiries with the neighbours or other parents. A childminder who is very obliging to you may be just as open hearted to everyone and regularly have far more children than her quota. If the house is immaculate, the children may have little opportunity to play. If the house is untidy, you must decide if this is acceptable clutter or a health and safety hazard. This should become obvious after a visit or two. However, a childminder may refuse to have children when they are ill – and young children can often have tummy upsets, bad coughs and mysterious rashes which could be infectious. Remember that you will have to fit in with her rather than expecting her to do what you want, so it is important to find someone with the same approach to childcare as yourself.

Day nurseries
Local-authority day nurseries have very few places for babies and these are usually allocated to single parents in severe financial or

social difficulties. Private nurseries, which may only take children who are toilet trained, have to be registered with the local authority, so you can find out from the council offices if there are any in your area. They are likely to have long waiting lists so it is important to put your name down early.

Day nurseries can seem an attractive option because they offer a stable environment and you are less likely to be 'let down'. However, they may be strict about not accepting children when they are ill.

Nannies and mother's helps

Trained nannies are expensive and do not do any general household duties, such as cooking your evening meal or doing the ironing. Many nannies and employers nowadays have contracts which spell out what is expected on both sides. You can, however, feel confident about leaving a young baby in their care. Nannies may live in your home or they may live out. If the nanny lives in, you are responsible for her welfare and if she is a long way from home she may be lonely at first. If she lives out, make sure that she will be able to arrive punctually. It is also worth checking with her referees about the state of her health. Will she, for example, soldier on with a cold, or expect to take to her bed at the slightest sniffle?

The expense can be eased if you share a nanny with another family, though with more children to look after she will expect to earn more from such an arrangement.

Mother's helps are not professionally trained. If they are not experienced, you will have to judge how well they will cope with routine duties and in an emergency.

One drawback with nannies and mother's helps is that they tend to change jobs fairly frequently, particularly if they are in an area where their services are in demand. A nanny who wants to leave after a year or 18 months is a problem because your child will have formed an attachment to her. It may help if you employ her for a trial period and agree to review the situation at the end of a year. This way you will feel more prepared to find someone new or to agree a change in her work practice, such as allowing her to take on more children so that she continues to feel stimulated.

Child swaps

Some women manage to arrange a regular swap with each other's children. This can seem an ideal solution, though probably is most successful if you work no more than 1½ days a week so that you have another 1½ days looking after the other child and two free days. Less free time than this can be a burden unless you are both single mothers, in which case sharing the childcare can be an added support – particularly if one of you falls ill.

KEEPING FIT

Being aware of your body will help you respond to the way it adapts to pregnancy and childbirth. Good posture and regular exercise will improve your muscle tone, relieve aches and pains and make you more supple.

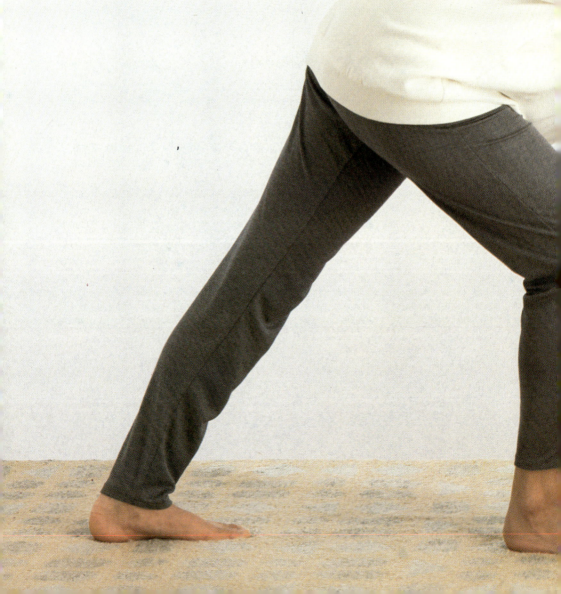

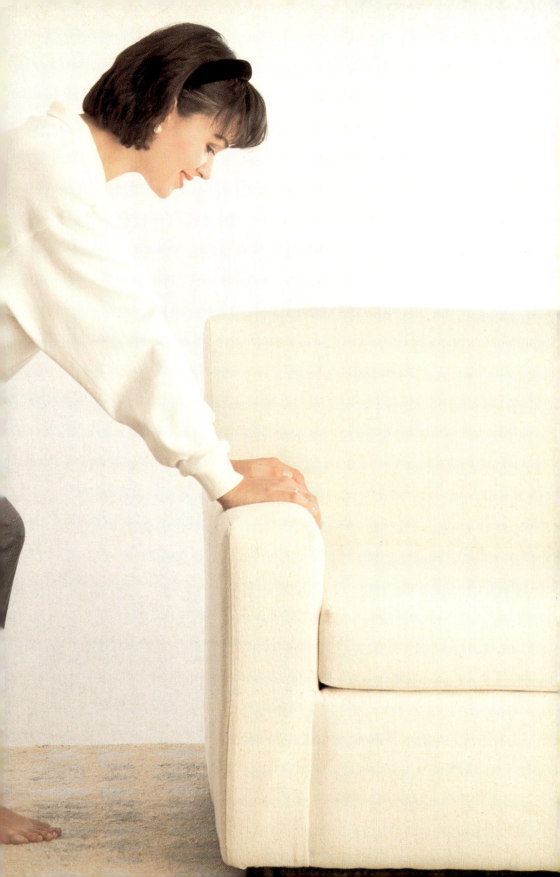

EVERYDAY
≈ *ACTION* ≈

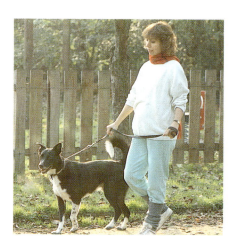

*D*uring pregnancy you probably feel more aware of your body and the way it is changing than at any time since puberty. Observing these changes and understanding how and why they are taking place is a wonderful foundation for building confidence as you discover your strengths and your limitations. There is no doubt you will cope better with looking after the physical demands of a baby if you are in good shape. Although pregnancy is not the time to go on an intensive training course without expert supervision, you can improve your suppleness, stamina and strength. In fact your body is adapting and becoming 'fitter' to quite a remarkable degree. But these changes also have their disadvantages and you may feel more aches and tiredness than before. You will need to make allowances for your softened ligaments and your altered balance of weight by not staying in the same position for long periods and taking more care about how you do household tasks. If you treat your body with care the drawbacks need not spoil this exciting time.

Giving up smoking

The female body has evolved to protect the developing fetus and, when functioning normally, is well able to provide all a baby needs for her growth and development. However what the body finds harder to do is to protect the baby from certain poisons such as cigarette smoke, alcohol (see page 45) and many drugs.

Nicotine stimulates the production of oxytocin, the labour hormone, and may induce premature labour. It also constricts the blood supply to the placenta so less oxygen gets through to the baby. Smoking or breathing in cigarette smoke therefore increases the chances of a baby being born premature, undernourished (because nutrients are also restricted) and with breathing problems. And a baby who continues to breathe in smoke after she is born will be more susceptible to chest and ear complications after a cough or cold. Once you know you are pregnant, make every effort to cut down and to give up by the fourth month of pregnancy; in this way your baby should be free of any possible effects. If you cannot give up, at least cut down as much as you can.

If you and your partner want to stop smoking – and do enlist his help if you both smoke – work out *why* you smoke. Understanding why, and when, you need a cigarette can help you give up. Is it because a cigarette acts like a marker for the different stages of your day? Is it a prop when you start a phone conversation? Is it to signal a change-over from work to relaxation? Is it to claim time for yourself? Is it to cope with meeting a deadline? Does nervousness make you want to fiddle with something? Working out what prompts you to smoke will help you find other distractions or ways of changing your behaviour patterns.

Cigarettes are addictive not only because of the nicotine they contain but also because they can relieve anxiety. There are other ways to get the same effect; see the breathing and relaxation techniques on pages 90–7. If you need the support of others, your antenatal clinic or the organization ASH (Action on Smoking and Health), see page 125, should be able to tell you where your nearest support group is.

'I so wanted to be "normal" again and do everything I did before I was pregnant that I was really quite shocked by how weak I felt if I rushed around. And I never expected so much backache from bending over.'

61

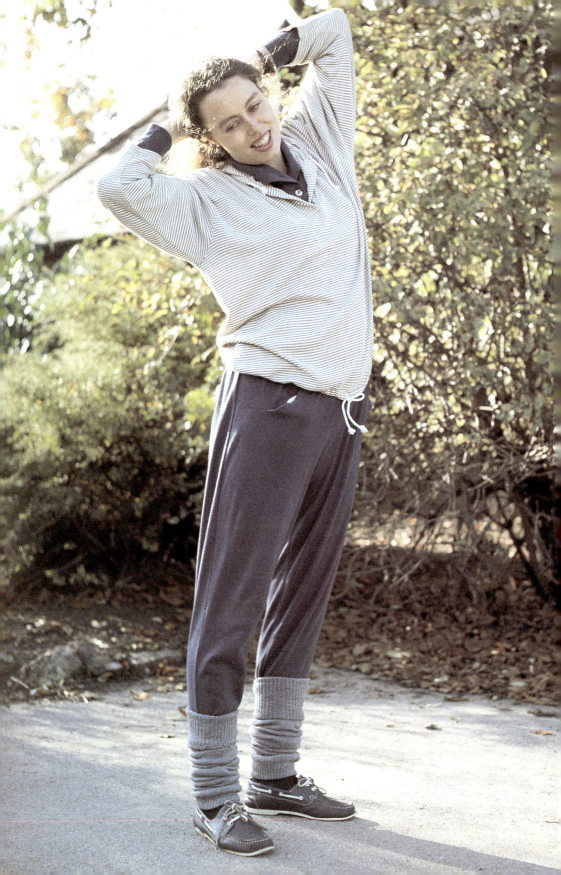

How your body adapts

Blood There is often a slowing down of the circulation and hence a lowering of blood pressure, resulting in lightheadedness and tiredness in the early weeks. But the volume increases by about 30–50 per cent during pregnancy. This increase and changes to the size of blood vessels near the surface of the skin may make you feel warmer. Increased weight and relaxing hormones may cause the veins of the legs and vulva to become varicose or swollen.

Heart By the seventh month the heart has grown larger and is working 40 per cent harder to pump the extra blood around. The growing uterus pushes it higher in the chest without any efficiency loss. You will feel no different and your pulse will hardly change.

Lungs Hormonal changes cause the breathing rate to increase so that up to 40 per cent more air is taken in. These physiological changes, together with the expanding uterus and bad posture, can cause breathlessness.

Ribcage Towards the end of pregnancy the ribs expand by as much as 7.5cm–10cm (3–4in) to allow for the growing uterus.

Abdominal muscles The two bands of muscle down the front of the body from chest to hip on either side of the navel can weaken and separate during pregnancy. Normally they meet in a slight hollow; after birth, they can be 2.5–15cm (1–6in) apart.

Digestive system Relaxing hormones cause the action of the digestive tract to slow down. The stomach may hold less during the last weeks of pregnancy if compressed by the expanding uterus.

Uterus (or womb) This bag of muscle grows in size five fold and its weight increases from about 50g (2oz) to 900g (2lb). It develops by means of contractions which happen spontaneously about every 20 minutes. After the birth, contractions, given extra stimulation by breastfeeding, help to shrink it to its former size.

Ligaments Relaxing hormones cause the fibrous tissue between bones to soften so that the body, and especially the pelvic area, becomes more flexible. This continues for three to five months after the birth. Bad posture and the weight of the growing uterus, as well as lifting and bending after the baby is born, can strain the ligaments anchoring the uterus to the spine and pelvis, causing backache.

Bladder The kidneys expand to hold six times more urine. In early pregnancy, before the body adapts, extra water is passed. In the last few weeks a frequent need to pass water can be caused by pressure from the uterus on the bladder.

Leg muscles The muscles of the legs and thighs strengthen and develop to carry the increasing weight. Cramps may be caused by slow circulation and the legs staying in one position for too long.

Learning good posture

Good posture helps prevent backache and makes you feel more confident. It also contributes to good muscle tone and lifts your ribs and chest so that you are able to breathe more easily. Because the ligaments are softened by hormonal changes during pregnancy, it is all too easy to thrust your tummy forward to maintain your centre of balance. Bad posture simply puts strain on the ligaments which are coping with the weight of the uterus and baby, weakens muscles and can become 'learned' so that after the birth you still sag.

Standing well

Take off your shoes and stand with your feet about hip width apart and only slightly turned out. Grasp the hair at the crown of your head and pull back and upwards. Feel the back of your neck and then the rest of your body – spine, backs of the thighs and knees – stretching and lengthening until your feet take your weight evenly. Once your balance is right, check your shoulders are dropped.

Sitting well

Sit with your knees about hip width apart in an upright chair with a small cushion or rolled towel behind the waist. Avoid crossing your legs as this twists the spine. If you have to sit for long, get up and stretch every half hour or do leg and ankle exercises (see page 76).

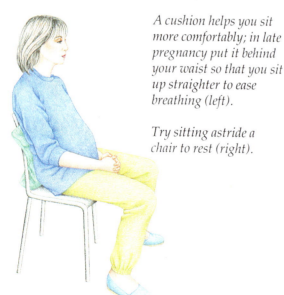

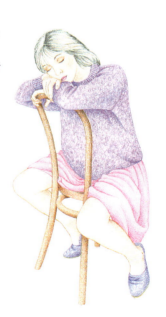

A cushion helps you sit more comfortably; in late pregnancy put it behind your waist so that you sit up straighter to ease breathing (left).

Try sitting astride a chair to rest (right).

Feeling tired

Sit astride an upright chair, facing the back, and support your chest with a cushion or your folded arms against it. Or kneel on the floor facing the seat of a soft chair, a pile of cushions or a bean bag, with your head resting on your arms. In these ways your back can be straight and your lungs free while you support much less of your body weight. If you are really tired, lie on your side with your top knee pulled up and comfortably supported with a pillow so that your back is completely straight and the weight of your body seems to fall away from your spine.

Lying down

You should not lie flat on your back for long: the weight of your uterus on your spine can slow down the blood supply to the placenta, making you feel sick or faint. The body is usually able to compensate for this in pregnancy, but lying on your back in labour can interfere with the contractions. If you want to relax on your back, lie with your head and upper back supported and a cushion under your knees to prevent your legs pulling on the abdominal muscles.

Getting out of bed

Always roll onto your side and use your arms to push yourself up from a lying position so that you put less strain on your weaker abdominal muscles and the softened ligaments in your spine.

Housework

Your ligaments and muscles will be soft and weak from early in pregnancy, and for a few months after the birth; these tips will help.

Washing-up Do it in short bursts rather than a lot at once.

Ironing Try using rhythmical movements, rocking your weight sideways from one foot to the other. If necessary, raise the ironing board or lower it and sit down.

Cleaning the bath Kneel on the floor and either lean forward or sideways; use a long-handled brush.

Vacuuming Turn it into a soothing, rhythmical rocking exercise – rocking backwards and forwards on your feet.

Tidying the floor Squat or have one knee on the floor and one knee raised, alternating knees as you work.

Going up stairs When you are heavily pregnant, you can take the weight off your legs and back by going on all fours.

Lifting a toddler (or heavy weight) Bend your knees and keep your back straight. If you can safely help your toddler to climb onto a low chair or bed, pick her up from there. Rather than stand, seat a toddler on a worktop for a cuddle.

After the baby is born

Your ligaments and muscles will take a few months to regain their normal elasticity and strength so you still need to take care after the baby is born. If it is your first child, or a long time since you last gave birth, your muscles will probably also need to get used to more lifting, carrying and bending.

Feeding positions
In the early weeks feeding will take up most of your waking hours. An incorrect position may not only mean that your nipples become increasingly sore but, if you are hunched or your muscles are tensed in one position, you may well get anxious, which will interrupt the milk flow besides giving you aching muscles and joints. You can feed sitting up or lying on your side. The latter position is useful after a Caesarean, if you have painful stitches or if you want to doze with your baby in the crook of your arm.

If you feed sitting up, you will probably find it easier in a firmly upholstered, upright chair with a cushion behind your waist, your knees bent and raised a little, perhaps with your feet resting on a stool. You may need a pillow or two across your lap to bring the baby up to breast height or to protect a Caesarean wound. Finally, making sure your baby's chest is facing yours, think about releasing any muscles which are tensing up in your neck, shoulders and arms.

If you feed lying on your side, position yourself so that you have

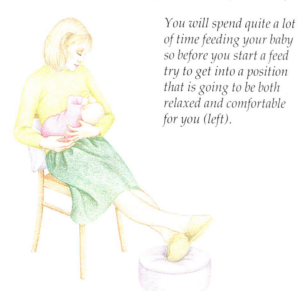

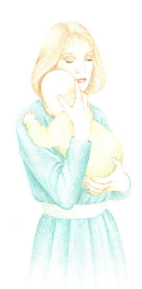

You will spend quite a lot of time feeding your baby so before you start a feed try to get into a position that is going to be both relaxed and comfortable for you (left).

your nipple level with your baby's top lip and wedge a rolled towel behind her back to stop her rolling away from you.

Lifting, bending and carrying
When lifting your baby out of a pram or cot, bend your knees and keep your back straight. Avoid leaning over and curving your spine.

The more you can do at waist height or higher, the more comfortable your back will be. Since nappy changes take place several times a day, it will help if you work at a convenient height.

Carry your baby with your back as straight as possible and your shoulders relaxed. She will probably enjoy being held upright, looking over your shoulder. When you are sitting, your baby may prefer being cradled with her back against your stomach looking out at the world.

Pelvic-floor exercises
While you are in hospital, you will be shown some gentle exercises, including those for the pelvic floor (see page 00). Ideally, they should be done at least four times every waking hour or every time you feed after the first couple of days until you no longer leak urine if you cough, sneeze or lift up your baby. This can take a few months. At first you may not be able to feel the pelvic-floor muscles, in which case you will need to practise pulling in the muscles of your rectum. These exercises are essential unless you take some other form of regular exercise. If you took plenty of exercise before the birth, you should find that you quickly regain control of your pelvic floor.

Your baby will enjoy being carried in this position; try to keep your back as straight as possible and relax your shoulders (left).

You may need to catch up with your sleep whenever you can so take the opportunity to doze when you have your baby blissfully curled up on your chest (left).

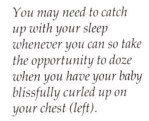

SPORT AND
≈ LEISURE ≈

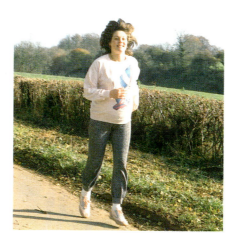

*P*regnancy can produce similar effects on the body's metabolism and physiology to vigorous exercise. The heart and circulation become automatically much more effective, and the softening of the ligaments allows much more flexibility and mobility in the joints.

Since the body is improving naturally, most doctors do not lay much emphasis on the need for extra exercise. But if you already enjoy activities like jogging, tennis, swimming, cycling, yoga or dancing, there is no reason you should not continue with all of them, provided you take some commonsense precautions. You should be aware that your ligaments are softening and your muscle tone is changing even before you start to look pregnant so be careful not to push yourself too hard and avoid any sudden movements. Highly competitive sports are not a good idea, if only because the desire to do well may stop you from listening to what your body is telling you.

Falls are more common in later pregnancy, when your centre of balance is altered. If you do fall, you are unlikely to hurt the baby, unless you receive a sharp blow to the abdomen, but you may easily damage yourself. Any activity for which a sense of balance and timing are essential and for which you need all your wits about you if you are to come to no harm should obviously not be undertaken in the last three months of pregnancy.

Improving muscle tone

Although extra exercise may not be strictly necessary during pregnancy, it can have a good effect on morale as well as helping to improve the strength of all your muscles. And without exercise all the good effects of pregnancy will wear off after the birth if they are not reinforced and maintained.

If you do decide to take more exercise, choose an activity in which you feel safe and take it slowly. Swimming, yoga and dancing are all excellent and safe forms of exercise. Not only do they improve all-round fitness, but they can help you enjoy your body more. They are also an excellent preparation for labour as well as teaching you ways to relax, essential if you are to make the most of the changes the new baby will bring to your life. But, as with all new activities, they should be approached with care. You will be exercising at the right pace if you find the activity easy, enjoyable and painless. Keep taking rests and build up slowly, stopping before you tire. A steady approach will help to keep your interest, ensuring that it soon becomes part of your way of life.

Activity	Stamina	Suppleness	Strength
Badminton	**	*	*
Climbing stairs	**	—	*
Cycling	***	*	**
Disco dancing	**	***	—
Housework	—	*	—
Jogging	***	*	*
Mowing the lawn	*	—	**
Squash	***	*	*
Swimming	**	**	***
Tennis	*	**	*
Walking briskly	**	—	*
Yoga	—	***	*

'I swam six lengths. I rested between each length but it was still six lengths. If I'd tried to swim without stopping, I would have exhausted myself after two and a half.'

Swimming

Swimming helps improve the efficiency of the heart, so increasing stamina, and by stretching the muscles and rotating the joints it also increases suppleness and strength. It is a particularly safe way of loosening up because the water provides support against the forces of gravity and prevents you from executing any sudden movements which could pull a muscle or ligament. When you are pregnant, being in the water can also be a special pleasure because of the sense of weightlessness and freedom it gives. You may find that there are swimming classes especially for pregnant women in your area.

Despite your increasing size, you will probably find you actually are more buoyant because of the extra fat you have gained. But exercise in water can be deceptive. If you are not used to swimming, you may find if you swim until you feel tired you have done too much. If you want to swim lengths, backstroke or sidestroke may be more comfortable than breaststroke, which can put a strain on your back if your neck is arched high.

After the birth swimming is an activity which both you and your baby can enjoy; it is excellent play for him and a good confidence-builder. It is best not to start until he has had his first immunizations (at three months) and your ligaments are returning to normal, but you should still take it gently at first. And, if you go with someone else so that you can share the baby minding, it can give you a much-needed opportunity for sociable exercise.

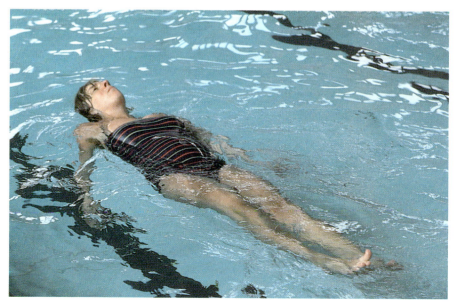

Water exercises

You can do more than just swim in a pool. The rail at the side provides an ideal barre for holding onto while you do stretching and curling exercises. You should also use the opportunity to maintain a steady breathing pattern and to become aware of releasing muscle tension as you breathe out.

Good movements to make while facing the rail are: swinging your legs from side to side; pushing off with your feet, and floating on your back for a minute or two while you keep your breathing calm and steady; curling your legs up and stretching them down again; and gently stretching your legs wide apart with your feet against the side. With your back to the rail, you can try holding on with your outstretched arms while doing bicycling movements with your legs or while pulling up your knees, opening your legs sideways and stretching them down before repeating the sequence.

You can, of course, invent your own exercises. Try to create sequences in which you can enjoy gradual stretching sensations and alternate bending or curling with opening-out movements.

Dancing

Dancing to music you love is an enjoyable and fun way of getting fit and an excellent preparation for labour contractions. Some rhythms can also be soothing.

Have two or three tapes of music with different rhythms so you can choose the one which suits your needs best and make up your own repertoire of arm and leg stretches, bends and circular movements. Sudden, jerky or forced movements can strain your pregnant body and may aggravate nausea in the early months so it is best to use music with a fairly steady beat. Slow, gentle music can aid concentration and relaxation, and the repetition of a phrase is also soothing, which is why a favourite song can be helpful. Fast, loud music can help relieve pain and has even been useful during labour.

Particularly good movements for pregnancy are: pelvic rocking actions – side to side, backwards and forwards, and in a circle clockwise and anticlockwise; arm stretches which open out your ribcage, particularly if the baby is pressing painfully on your ribs; and gentle, circular swings, moving your arms from side to side to loosen the shoulders and neck muscles. If you feel unsure of your balance, hold the back of a heavy chair with one hand.

After the birth you can dance with your baby. He will love the rocking, rhythmical movements as well as the sound of the music. You can also gently stretch and move your baby's arms and legs in time to the rhythm, as well as tapping out the beat on his body.

Yoga

Yoga can help you improve your body's suppleness and poise while teaching you greater self-awareness. With practice and the correct breathing techniques, it can be deeply relaxing for the mind and the body, bestowing an inner peace and serenity which is wonderful for building your self-confidence. It is almost as if yoga were devised for the pregnant woman with her improved lung capacity and softened ligaments.

Yoga exercises are based on the principle of alternating cycles of muscle tension with periods of relaxation, while maintaining the rhythm of breathing slowly in and out. It is essential to begin practising yoga with an experienced teacher; you may be able to find a special yoga-for-pregnancy class near you. You need guidance because although yoga requires people to work within their own

*BADDHA
KONASANA*

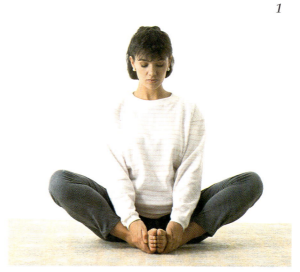

1

Sit on the floor with your legs together, stretched straight in front of you. Bend your knees and, keeping them together, bring your feet as close to your body as possible. Place the soles and heels of your feet together so that the outside edges are resting on the floor and grasp your toes.

Pull your feet inward as close to the perineum as you comfortably can, keeping your elbows straight and letting your knees open outwards until they are as near to the floor as possible (1).

Stretch your spine upwards and hold this position for as long as is comfortable, all the time breathing steadily in and out through your nose.

Place your elbows on your thighs and, bending your elbows, press downwards until you begin to feel the pull on the inner thighs. Breathe out, bending forward as far as you can, and hold the position for 30–60 seconds, feeling the stretch but keeping the

breathing steady. (An experienced yogi can get her knees, chin and nose to touch the floor!)

Breathe in as you raise yourself slowly into the upright position, bring your knees together and straighten your legs so that you resume the starting position.

limitations and to extend these boundaries gradually, it demands considerable self-discipline to do so. Unfortunately, too many of us are either too impatient, lazy or competitive so that we push ourselves too hard or get bored, complaining of too little stimulation.

After the birth, if you already practise yoga, you can restart gently in about the fifth week and from three months you can resume your normal level.

The poses or asanas illustrated here have been particularly recommended for pregnancy and as a preparation for labour. The yoga teacher B.K.S. Iyengar said of Baddha Konasana or the Indian cobbler position: 'It is found that pregnant women who sit daily in this pose for a few minutes will have much less pain during delivery and will be free from varicose veins.' The poses can be hard work so you need a few minutes of complete relaxation after a session (see page 90). Throughout all yoga poses it is very important to keep the breathing steady.

UPAVISTHA KONASANA

2

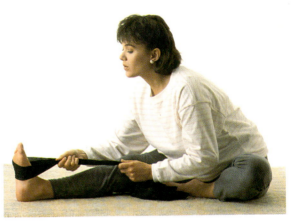

Sit on the floor with your legs together stretched straight in front of you. Move each leg sideways until they are as far apart as possible, making sure that the whole of each leg is resting on the floor.

Grasp your toes (if you can't reach them, loop a scarf round each foot) and, keeping your spine straight, pull the upper part of your body forward and downward towards the floor. Stay in this position for 30–60 seconds, keeping your breathing steady. Then, as you breathe in, release your feet, bring your legs together and relax.

If this is too difficult, you may find the following modified version easier.

Sit with both your legs stretched out and bend one knee. Draw that foot up as close to the perineum as possible. Loop a scarf round the extended foot and, keeping your spine straight, pull your body forward and as close to that knee as you can (2).

Release your foot and breathe in as you raise your back to an upright position. Straighten your bent knee to resume the starting position.

Repeat, bending the other knee. Finally, bring your legs together, straighten up and rest for a few moments.

≈ *EXERCISE* ≈

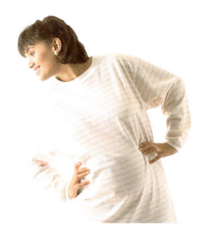

*E*xercise is important in three ways: it increases strength, suppleness and stamina; it makes you feel good; and it is an excellent
way of relieving the effects of stress and aiding relaxation. Obviously,
the exercise habit is good for your health. Unfortunately finding the
opportunity for exercise is not that easy. It isn't just laziness that
makes us opt for the car or bus rather than walking. Cars and buses
save time – and time is precious. So, unless exercise can be fitted in as
some part of an existing activity, it tends to be neglected. Doing just a
few exercises whenever you can is helpful and if the presence of
other people is inhibiting, you can probably do fairly discreet
stretching, shaking and circular movements to stimulate and relax
any muscles which have grown tense and uncomfortable after being
fixed in one position for any length of time.

Babies and children often encourage their parents to take more
exercise. If being taken out in the pram keeps the baby amused or
sends her off to sleep, then mothers will be glad to find time to go for
walks, and if running around or a game of football in the park uses
up some of the children's surplus energy, then parents will enjoy the
shared fun and fitness.

But if you are pregnant for the first time, finding the opportunity
for exercise can seem an added burden and the idea of a 20-minute

routine will probably not fill you with enthusiasm. It is worth remembering the following: new mothers often complain they have no time for themselves because every waking moment is spent lavishing care on the baby; looking after a baby is physically demanding because your muscles have to get used very quickly to different ways of working; the lack of a structure for each day is one of the most disorientating things about new motherhood and most mothers feel more secure with some kind of routine, whether or not their babies mind; and lastly, doing exercises with your baby is an excellent way of keeping you both happy, important because your confidence can be a little fragile at first, when the change in your life is a shock, whether you are enjoying it or finding things hard.

The most important thing about exercise is to make it an integral part of your life, like brushing your teeth. Exercise classes, such as you may attend in pregnancy, can be a wonderful way of making new friends and an excellent boost at the beginning if you are particularly low on willpower or if you find group support a real help. But as a way of taking exercise they tend to be a temporary rather than a permanent feature of life for most people. You need to concentrate on finding ways that will keep exercise a part of your lifestyle. In the pages which follow, the exercises do not have to be done as part of a routine. For example, foot and ankle exercises can be done sitting in a bus, squatting can be practised when on the phone at home, curl-ups before getting out of bed, the yoga positions while watching television, and pelvic tilts on all fours tidying the floor. Even if you have a demanding toddler, or are tied to a desk all day, you can refresh yourself with a few warm-up and stretching exercises every now and again. Taking care of your body in these small ways will help prevent fatigue and frustration so that you feel fitter and will probably be inspired to take more demanding forms of exercise more often!

'I sometimes have to force myself to go to the exercise class, but I'm always glad when I've been. I feel really relaxed and peaceful, not exhausted and drawn as I do after a day of just sitting in the office.'

Warming-up

Warming-up exercises have three important functions: they stimulate the circulation, preparing the heart for pumping harder; they cause the cartilage in the joints to thicken by as much as 50 per cent, making the joints stronger and less liable to injury, and they 'heat up' the muscles, increasing their elasticity and power as they call up more energy from the body's reserves. Warming-up is like an injection of fitness and energy. If you don't warm up before exercise, you are more likely to suffer cramp, stiffness and injury.

FEET AND ANKLES
*Stretch your toes and then curl them (**1**). Raise your feet a couple of inches and rotate your ankles (**2**) clockwise and anticlockwise. Again with your feet raised, point your toes and then push down your heels.*

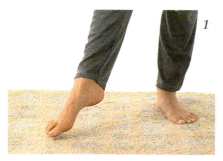

1

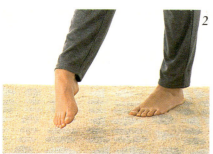

2

PELVIS AND SPINE
*Clench and then relax your buttock muscles. Pull up your pelvic floor and then push it down. Push your hips forward and back. With your hands on your hips, bend sideways from the waist, straighten up and twist to look behind you (**3**). With feet just apart, hold onto something steady, bend the knees a little and lean forwards from the waist. Straighten your legs and then bend them again as you come up.*

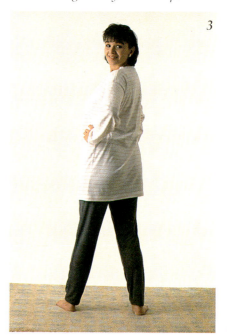

3

LEGS
Shake each leg from the knee. Holding onto a shelf or something sturdy, bend your knees and then straighten them. Stretch and shake each leg from the hip.

It is important to warm up all the muscles in the body because they are all used. It doesn't matter where you start, but it is probably easier if you begin either from your feet or your face. Do each movement three or four times very gently and only take bending and twisting movements as far as feels comfortable.

You can warm up different parts of the body for a couple of minutes at intervals during the day. Try, for example, exercising your face and neck while watching television, or your shoulders and arms every time you get up after sitting for long periods. Doing a few gentle exercises frequently will help keep your muscles loose, release tension and reduce fatigue.

SHOULDERS AND ARMS

*Shrug your shoulders up (**4**) and then pull them down (**5**). Draw your shoulder blades back simultaneously and then curl your shoulders towards the front. Circle each shoulder clockwise and anticlockwise, keeping the other shoulder still as you do so. Stretch your arms, hands and fingers out sideways, release them and feel the warmth of the relaxed muscles, and then shake them.*

NECK AND FACE

*Bend your chin down onto your chest (**6**) and then bend back, pulling up the jaw (**7**). Bend your neck from side to side towards your shoulders. Turn your neck slowly round to look behind, then back and to the other side. Open your mouth as wide as possible sideways and then up and down to stretch the facial muscles. Raise and then lower your eyebrows. Gently rub your face and brow with your hands.*

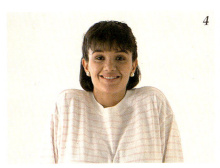

4

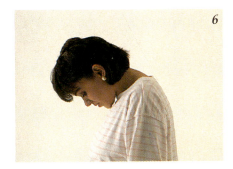

6

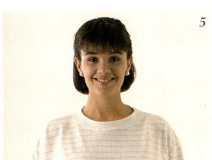

5

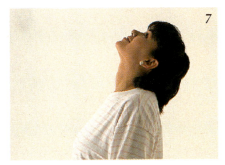

7

Early and middle pregnancy

*T*hese more demanding exercises are meant to be done when your muscles are already loosened up after the warm-up routine, or some rough and tumble with your toddler or, indeed, any physical activity which has left you feeling fit and ready for more.

THE SQUAT

Squatting stretches and strengthens the muscles of the pelvic floor, lower back and legs.

Stand with your feet slightly more than hip width apart, toes forward, and hold onto a stable object. Gradually lower your bottom until you are squatting comfortably with your feet flat on the floor. Hold for 10 seconds, longer as your balance gradually improves.

To help keep your feet flat, press your back against a wall as you lower yourself. Or with your heels raised, use your hands to balance you (*1*).

When you can squat easily, point your toes slightly sideways and, clasping your hands, push with your elbows against your inner thighs for 30–60 seconds. Increase the pressure as your thigh muscles strengthen. Stop before the backs of your knees feel uncomfortable and don't bounce in a squat. Straighten your legs afterwards to take any strain off your joints.

1

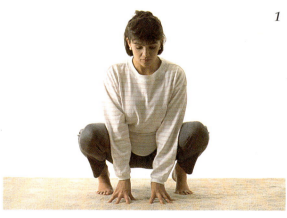

CURL-UPS

2

Curl-ups strengthen the abdominal muscles.

☐ Lie on your back with your head and shoulders on a firm cushion, your legs together. Bend your knees and, placing your arms across your abdomen, pull the stomach muscles together as you lift your head and shoulders (*2*). Hold the position for up to 10

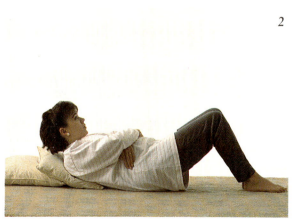

seconds, longer if you can, and then relax. Support your abdomen or you may simply push the muscles further apart.

SPINE STRETCHERS
Because the ligaments in the back and pelvis soften and the hip joints get much looser during pregnancy many women suffer pain in the lower back. These exercises stretch the muscles. If one side of your back is already painful, raise the knee on that side and do the following exercises to give the affected part of the back a gentle stretch.
□ Lie on your back with your legs together. Bend one knee up as far as you can and take hold of that foot with your opposite hand so that the foot points towards the opposite hip (**3**). Gently pull the knee and then relax. Repeat several times; then do the same with the other leg.
□ Lie on your back with your legs together. Bend one knee up until you can tuck the foot under the outside of the opposite calf (**4**). Gently twist and roll the bottom of your spine towards the bent knee, keeping your shoulders flat (**5**). Repeat with the other leg.

The two yoga positions on pages 72–3 are also excellent for strengthening the back, thighs and pelvic floor.

3

4

5

Later pregnancy

*I*n the last two months of pregnancy you will be thinking more about the actual birth and how to prepare for it and, in the final weeks, your baby will be trying to settle into a comfortable delivery position. During the birth, first of all the muscle contractions of the uterus will be opening up the cervix. Later on, you use your diaphragm and abdominal muscles to help your uterus bear down while releasing your pelvic-floor muscles to let the baby out. The more you can follow your body's sensations through those stages, the more you can help yourself. The following exercises will help prepare your body for the physical action of giving birth.

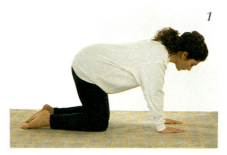

1

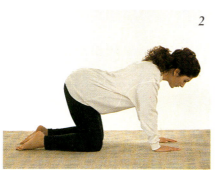

2

ABDOMINAL AND BACK EXERCISES

*Go down on all fours with your knees hip width apart and your hands shoulder width apart. Tilt your pelvis smoothly backwards and forwards so that the small of the back is arched (**1**) and then slightly hollowed (**2**). Don't hollow the back too much or you risk straining it.*

*Start as above; rotate your hips in a circular movement a few times, then rock gently backwards (**3**) and forwards (**4**) and then from side to side in a smooth, gentle rhythm. This can be a soothing exercise in labour and some midwives believe that taking the weight of the uterus away from the spine, in the last six weeks of pregnancy, enables the baby to get into a better position.*

3

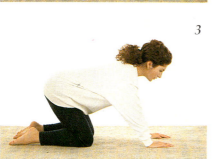

4

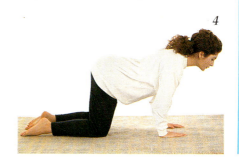

DIAPHRAGM EXERCISES

The diaphragm helps the uterus bear down in the second stage of pregnancy. You can feel this muscle action if you press your lips to the side of your fist and blow (**5**). As your cheeks balloon, you should be able to feel your diaphragm bearing down and your pelvic floor bulging out. You can practise this action and teach yourself how to recognize precisely how your muscles act when they are bearing down every time you open your bowels.

Breathing should be deep for any sustained, vigorous activity, such as labour (see page 94). Practise slow, deep breathing when you exercise and be aware of your abdomen pushing out as you breathe in and subsiding as you breathe out (**6**).

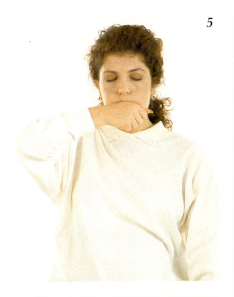

5

PELVIC-FLOOR EXERCISES

Lie on your back with your knees drawn up (**7**) and gradually pull in the muscles between your legs as if you were trying to prevent your bladder emptying. Hold the muscles for up to 10 seconds, relax and finally push them out so that they bulge and let go. Don't pull in the muscles suddenly or you will only strengthen a few instead of all the muscles of the pelvic floor.

You can check if you are pulling these muscles effectively by stopping the stream of urine half way through emptying your bladder. If you can do this easily, your muscles are working well. That is the level of efficiency you need to try to regain after the birth. But while you are pregnant, it is more important to stretch those muscles by bulging them out (as when you blow on your fist). Practise during squatting (see page 78) and when sitting with your legs wide apart.

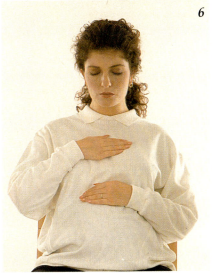

6

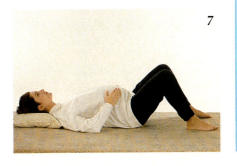

7

What happens in a normal labour

*L*abours are individual experiences that can vary for one woman with each baby she has. Some labours build up gradually and a few start with a sudden burst of activity. First babies are usually, but by no means necessarily, born after longer labours. No suggestions or guidelines can be helpful for everyone. But anything which encourages you to 'tune into' your body so that you listen to it and follow its lead will help you.

Towards the end of pregnancy many women experience spurts of contractions which, despite promising beginnings, do not develop into full labour. Knowing when labour has started can be a problem even for doctors and midwives, but much more important is knowing when labour is strongly established and will stay that way until the baby is born.

The purpose of pain
If pain has been something you have always been anxious to avoid, the idea that it can have a useful purpose may seem strange. However, it is an important concept to consider when you are going to have a baby as it can colour your whole attitude to labour.

Acute pain has an important biological function. It is part of the body's protective mechanism because it forces the sufferer to do something about it. If there were no pain during the birth process, babies could end up being born in unsuitable surroundings.

Pain also makes you gradually withdraw into yourself. This happens because your body is trying to make you listen to it so that you can find a way of comforting it. You may find relief by rubbing the sore place to stimulate the brain's production of endorphins, the body's natural painkillers, or by trying out different positions. This is all for your own and the baby's good: moving about and letting gravity pull on different parts of your body can help the baby move into a better birth position.

Pain is a very powerful way of calling for the help and support of others. Unfortunately we sometimes don't make the most of it. Too many of us have been schooled to ignore the demands of the body, believing that making helpful noises like groans and moans is rude and self-indulgent.

Pain is also a challenge, particularly when there is something joyful or fulfilling at the end of it. Remember the pain on the faces of marathon runners?

On the other hand, if pain is regarded as something that must be either 'suffered because it is deserved' or 'avoided at all costs', it is simply made worse because both attitudes ignore the body's call for help. Doing something to help yourself does not just mean being able to manage the labour on your own or with the support of others. It may also mean knowing when is the appropriate time to ask for pain relief or to accept some other medical assistance.

The stages of labour

□ At the beginning, if you can carry on with what you were doing during contractions and feel excited or happy and chatty between them, then the more you will enjoy this early stage. Restlessness in early labour is nature's way of warming up your muscles.

□ As the contractions become stronger, you will find it more difficult to 'just carry on' because you need to concentrate hard. At this point you will probably want the reassuring presence of your partner. Being upright and moving about in a rhythmical, rocking motion can not only be comforting but can also help open the cervix by causing the baby's head to press down onto it. If you are tired or want to be still, then lying in a warm, but not hot, bath can be soothing.

□ As the contractions become yet more powerful, you will find that you want to be where you are going to have your baby and with the people who are going to help you.

□ On arrival at hospital labour can sometimes cease as your body is put on alert because of new surroundings. The midwife will know your body needs to be undistracted which is why she may leave you in privacy for a while to help the labour get going again. But you can help

regain this concentration if you shut your eyes, listen to some music on a personal stereo and make noises and move about as restlessly as you like.

□ As labour progresses, if you are coping well your partner will notice you withdraw into yourself. Between contractions you may simply want to be quiet, either lying on your side or draped over a bean bag or the back of a chair or leaning over the bed, your feet on the floor.

□ Towards the end of the first stage the contractions may be so frequent and intense that you feel you have had enough and may even lose all interest in the baby. This is when the love, caresses, praise and encouragement of those with you will get you through what is for most women the worst part of labour.

□ At the end of the first stage everything sometimes slows down for a while and you can rest and prepare yourself for the contractions that will bring your baby into the world.

□ The second stage of labour is for many women simply hard, even enjoyable, work as they give three or four pushes – with maybe some satisfying grunts – during each contraction. Finally you will feel the elastic skin around your vagina stretching as your baby emerges.

Positions for labour and birth

*F*inding a comfortable position is the first step in helping you work with your contractions during labour. You do not have to be lying down or even sitting still. In fact, you may find being up and about, particularly in the early part of labour, very helpful.

Some of the positions you may find most helpful are not necessarily those which come easily to mind. Those into which you can introduce some rocking or circular movement of the hips are particularly helpful. And being upright makes it easier for you to shift your weight as well as allowing gravity to help pull the baby's head down onto the cervix. Remember too that beds are not just for lying on. You can kneel, leaning over the bed snuggled into lots of pillows. Or sit up with your legs hanging over the edge, or with one foot tucked underneath you, as you rock backwards and forwards or sideways, a particularly useful position if you have to have a drip tube inserted into a vein. But if you want to lie down and stay absolutely still, then lie on your side rather than on your back. Lying on your back lessens the blood supply to the uterus, interfering with the work of the contractions. Your partner can get on the bed behind you with his knees pulled up and you sitting cradled in between his legs with your arms around his knees. He can then stroke your brow, breasts or tummy or simply hold you. This is also a good position for giving birth as your partner's body will help prevent you from slipping down.

More important than adopting any position you may read about, is to shut your eyes and really listen to what *your* body wants. During labour it is working by means of a series of muscular contractions, first to make an opening from the uterus and then to push out the baby and later the placenta. Anything which helps you establish some kind of regular rhythm – whether it be rocking, stroking,

A position that can help to take any pressure from your back during labour is to kneel beside a bed leaning over it and supporting yourself comfortably on lots of pillows.

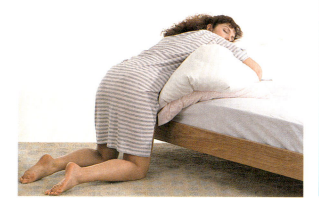

If you feel comfortable squatting, you may find it helpful to use the end of a bed for extra support.

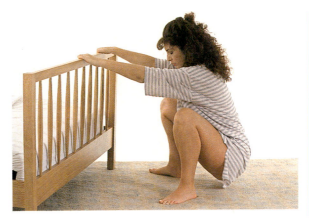

breathing or groaning – is likely to make it easier for you to work with each contraction. Never mind if you lose the rhythm. Just relax after the contraction and start again with the next one. If you are keen to have some form of pain relief, then soothing yourself with a rhythmical action will help keep your mind clear so that you can decide what to have and when to have it.

Birth positions

Any of the labour positions in which you are not sitting directly on your vagina can be used for giving birth, provided you feel secure and your midwife is happy. (If she has a bad back, she may not be too enthusiastic about squatting on the floor!)

Some hospitals have a birthing chair or a bed which can be fixed in an upright supporting position so that you can sit up more easily for delivery. If you do not express a preference and you are having a normal delivery, then you will probably be manoeuvred into a reclining squat. You can practise beforehand by pretending you are opening your bowels in this position. If it feels comfortable, fine. If not, you can roll over from this position onto one buttock (see below).

This well supported squatting position enables gravity to help the baby's head down and opens up the pelvic bones as well as avoiding sitting directly on the vagina and tail bone.

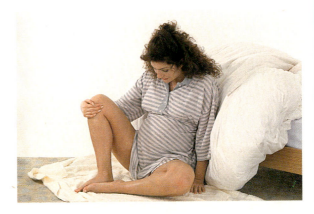

After the baby is born

Your tummy, legs and pelvic floor may feel rather weak in the first two days when you have to get up to go to the lavatory and to feed your baby. You will find getting up easier if you get the circulation going in your legs by doing some foot-warming exercises (see page 76). Then take a few slow abdominal breaths (see page 94) and, as you breathe out, feel your stomach muscles pulling in; hold and support your abdomen in this position as you draw up your knees and roll over to get out of bed. This preparation is particularly important if you have had a Caesarean.

To rest, lie on your front with a pillow under your tummy, and another under your breasts, or on your back with a pillow under your thighs, or on your side with a pillow under your breasts.

DAY THREE ONWARDS
Muscle weakness will cause you to feel tired but a few gentle exercises for the rest of the first week will help you gradually feel better.
☐ *Lie on your back, with your head and shoulders resting on a couple of pillows, bend up your knees and tilt your pelvis slightly backwards and forwards to help regain a good*

posture and to ease backache. You can also do some pelvic-floor exercises in this position (see page 81).
☐ *In the same position, tilt your pelvic floor until your waist touches the bed and then see how far you can slide your legs down before your back arches. (You may only manage a few inches at first but try every few hours and your abdominal muscles will*

regain their strength.)
☐ *Bring your knees up again and try raising your head and shoulders by pulling on your stomach muscles (1). Again, you may only manage an inch or two at first. If your tummy bulges and you cannot keep it braced, you are pushing yourself too fast.*

The warm-up exercises for neck, shoulders and arms will get rid of tension before and after feeding (see page 77).

1

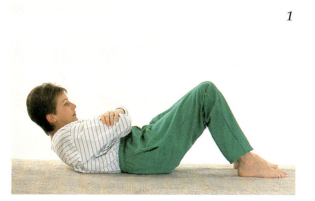

NEXT FEW WEEKS
You can begin some slightly more energetic exercises, though they still need to be gentle as your ligaments require careful treatment. Try to do the exercises twice a day and do each one three or four times, gradually building up to 20 times.

FINDING YOUR WAIST AGAIN

Sit well back on an upright chair with your spine straight and your knees and feet hip width apart. Breathe out, holding your tummy with one hand, and then bend sideways slowly (2). Repeat, bending to the other side. Fold your arms at shoulder level, slowly twist to look behind and then twist back. Drop gently forward from the waist; after 30–60 seconds straighten up slowly.
☐ *Lie on your back, bend your knees up together and lift your buttocks while pulling in your pelvic floor (3). Your trunk and thighs should form a straight line. Lower your body and, holding your ribs to keep your trunk straight, turn your knees to one side and then the other as far as is comfortable.*

AFTER SIX WEEKS

Incorporate more energetic exercises: lying on your side and raising the upper leg; on all fours, curling one leg up, stretching it out behind and then curling it back (4); and bottom shuffling along the floor.

Finish with a short relaxation (see page 90).

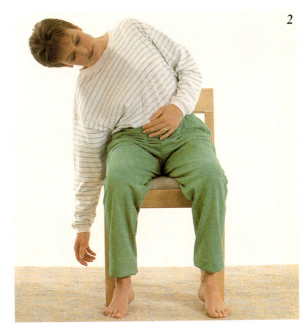

2

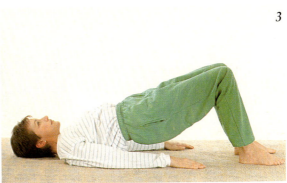

3

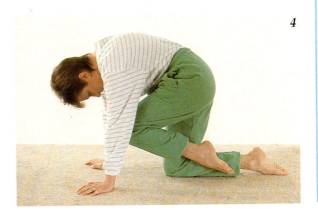

4

RELAXATION

Learning to relax your body will help you cope with labour and the early weeks of settling down with your baby. Massage is a very pleasurable aid to relaxation and can be enjoyed by you, your partner and your new baby.

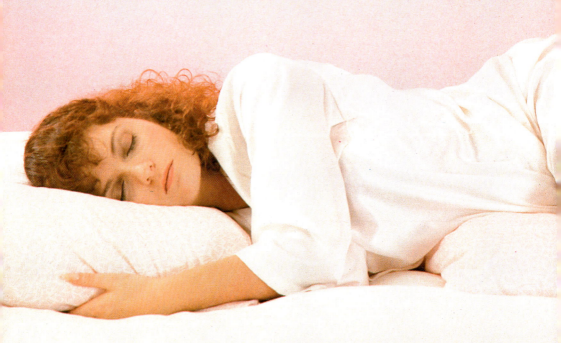

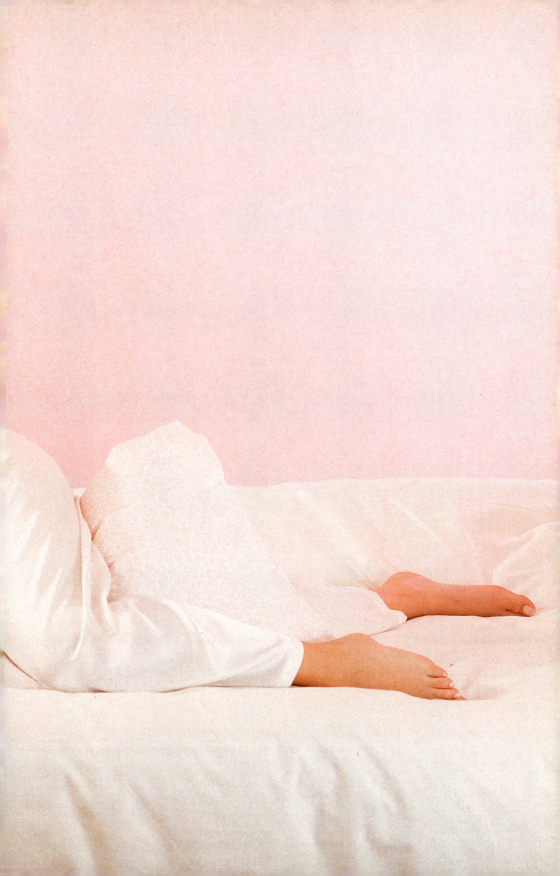

LEARNING
≈ TO UNWIND ≈

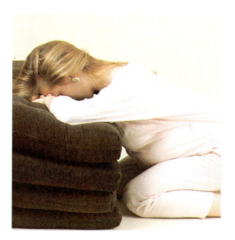

Relaxation often seems impossible – especially at those times when you need it most. This is perhaps not surprising when you realize that relaxing is very difficult unless you first understand just what stress and tension are. Knowing precisely what causes tension in you and how your body expresses it are essential if you are to learn how to relieve it.

When you are excited or under stress, whether it is pleasurable or painful, your body reacts in a special way. Muscles contract or tighten, ready for action, and hormones are released to give a burst of energy. Your breathing pattern is affected too as you instinctively take in more oxygen for the expected activity. But, if that energy is never called on and the muscles stay 'on the ready', you begin to feel tired, anxious and irritable. And if the oxygen is not used up, it causes a slight feeling of dizziness or faintness, which sets off your body's alarm system, causing a vicious circle of overbreathing.

Imagine yourself stuck in a traffic jam with an important appointment ahead of you. How does your body react? Are you leaning forward, willing the traffic to move? Do you clench the steering wheel or drum a tattoo upon it? Do you notice changes in your breathing patterns? Are there frequent sighs, fast breathing, deep inward breaths as if you cannot get enough air and even yawns?

Learning to relax

Once you are able to recognize the physical signs of tension in your body, you can make an effort to stretch and loosen muscles so that you 'wind down' instead of 'winding up'. Exerting physical control over your muscles has a calming effect on your emotions.

It is for this reason that exercise is such an excellent antidote to stress and tension: it converts surplus energy in ways which can refresh you. However, it is not always easy to conjure up the right circumstances for exercise, whereas relaxation techniques can be practised anytime. Learning relaxation has other benefits too. It eases aches and pains by changing the action of muscles; it can help lower blood pressure; it reduces tiredness; it increases your capacity to bear pain and it helps improve your relationships.

Using relaxation techniques will also help you *feel* good – by keeping your mind clear so that you can take stock of situations and assess priorities and by giving you greater self-awareness. Both are particularly valuable skills in pregnancy and the early days of parenthood, when you are likely to experience emotional highs and lows and when you have to work out what you can or cannot do.

At first, when you are learning to relax, you will need to find a quiet place where you can sit or lie comfortably. Later you can try relaxing while you are standing and then in situations which make you tense. If often helps to warm up first (see page 76).

Relaxation in labour

During labour, performing a relaxation technique between contractions is a very important way of coping with pain. Pain is always made worse by tension and waiting for the pain to come again: with increasing tension comes exhaustion, which in turn makes any pain worse. Learning to relax in labour will not only help you through contractions but will also let you enjoy the intervals between them. This will conserve your stamina and help keep your mind clear for decisions about the management of your labour.

'I really remember the relaxation I learned in antenatal classes but at the time I found it hard to take it seriously.'

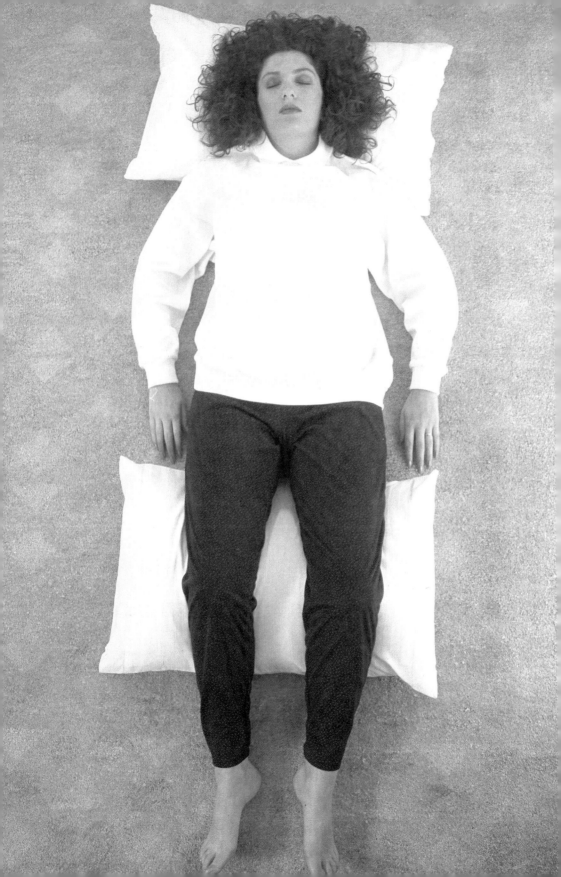

Whole-body relaxation

A sk someone to read the instructions below slowly in a calm, quiet voice or make a tape, leaving a 5-minute pause after instruction 17 and ending up with the suggestions for getting your muscles back into working order. You could use the tape on a personal stereo and, if possible, practise relaxation for 10 minutes on the bus or tube, travelling to work.

1. Get comfortable. Make sure your head and neck feel at ease. If you can, close your eyes. If not, focus on something not too far away. You are going to think about each part of your body in turn: notice how it feels after you have stretched and let go.

2. Start with your feet. Wriggle your toes, rotate the ankles and then let them drop.

3. Bend your feet up at the ankles, push your heels down and feel the stretch on the back of your calves and let go.

4. Roll your thigh muscles out and then let them go.

5. Let your bottom sink into the chair or floor.

6. Lengthen your spine. Imagine the bones in your back are a string of beads. Working from the tail bone up, try to make a space between each bead.

7. Stretch the back of your neck right up to the crown of your head. Imagine someone pulling a string attached to your crown, making the back of your neck feel long.

8. Now imagine your scalp. Try and 'feel' a space between each hair on your head.

9. Smooth out your forehead so the eyebrows are farther apart.

10. Let your cheeks feel soft.

11. Unclench your teeth and let your jaw drop. Make sure your tongue is away from the roof of your mouth.

12. Push your shoulders down and then let go.

13. Push your arms a little away from your sides and let them go.

14. Stretch your fingers and then let them go.

15. And just stay there. If a part of your body feels tense, then stretch and release it, feeling the difference. If your baby's kicking is distracting, stroke your tummy gently round and round to give yourself another rhythm to concentrate on.

16. To stop your mind from being distracted by any busy thoughts, fix your attention on the softness of the cushion you are leaning on or the hum of traffic going by.

17. Feel your breathing become steadier and rest for at least 1–2 minutes, 5 if you can.

18. Gradually start to pull your muscles together, gently bringing your circulation back to its usual pace. Open your eyes, look around and *when you are ready* have a big stretch and maybe a yawn.

Deep breathing

Y ou probably give little thought to the way you breathe until something happens to change it. For instance, in the last few weeks of pregnancy, when the baby may be pressing on your lungs, you may find yourself taking occasional gulps of air or heaving deep sighs. But even if you are not aware of your own breathing, you may have noticed how others breathe. The way a person breathes is a useful indication of how relaxed he or she is.

Anxiety causes the breathing to become shallow and rapid so that you can see the upper part of the chest moving. This overbreathing – or hyperventilation – often makes people feel as if they cannot get enough air so they put all their effort into taking air in rather than breathing it out. Eventually they feel 'muzzy', headachy or just plain tired because of the imbalance in the breathing mechanism. A relaxed person, on the other hand, has breathing which is hardly visible in the chest. Instead, the action takes place at the level of the abdomen. If you watch a child sleeping, you'll see the stomach rise with the inward breath and fall with the outward one.

Check your own breathing. Lie on the floor with your head and shoulders supported on a pillow and put a piece of paper on your chest and another at the base of your ribs above your diaphragm. Which piece of paper moves?

Learning the technique
Abdominal breathing can be learned, though when you are not used to it, it can feel strange at first. Lie down and breathe out to empty your lungs, then breathe in as much as you would normally but this time let the ball of air pass right down to the bottom of your lungs. This is 'deep' breathing: it's *not* filling the whole of the lungs with as much air as possible. Practise slow deep breathing three or four times, and pause a little between the breaths in and out.

Once you get used to deep, abdominal breathing, you should always think about the outward breath, letting it be calm and unhurried. You don't need to worry about the inward breath; that will look after itself. Try and practise when you feel anxious and discover how slow, deep breathing calms you down.

Unwinding in a hurry
Next time you are caught in a traffic jam or waiting to see someone who makes you feel nervous, try the following exercise. Push your shoulders down, stretch the muscles in your hands, arms, feet and jaw and release them. Then take two or three slow deep breaths, concentrating on letting out the outward breath. Make an effort to

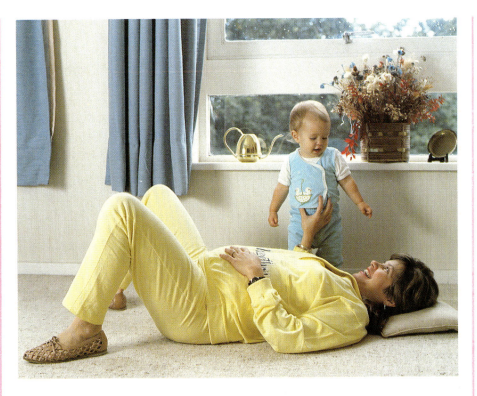

feel and notice the difference. As you get better at recognizing muscle tension before it really takes hold, you will find that you can 'let go' of your muscles without having to stretch them first.

Preparing for labour

During labour you may have to take bigger breaths than usual because your body will be working harder. In preparation you can practise keeping your breathing calm and unhurried through a simulated contraction.

Sit in the cobbler position (see page 72) and gradually push down with your elbows on the insides of your legs for 30 seconds; then slowly release the pressure for another 30 seconds. This mimics the build-up of a contraction, or tightening, of the uterus, reaching a peak and then slowly easing off. As you feel your muscles take the strain, you will have to concentrate harder to keep your breathing calm and unhurried.

Your breathing in labour will be faster too. Faster breathing usually means breathing with your mouth open, which can soon result in a dry mouth. So practise breathing in through your nose and out through your mouth. This may feel awkward when you are not exercising hard but it helps in labour.

Labour and after

*T*he body's automatic reaction to sudden discomfort or pain is to tense the muscles and hold the breath or gasp, preparing for what is commonly called 'flight or fight'. The strength of contractions during labour can often produce this response. If it continues, you and the baby will soon tire. The tension and irregular breathing pattern will make you anxious and confused so that you end up fighting the contractions instead of working with them.

Working with the contractions
You need to be able to release any tension which builds up during the contractions. The following technique will help.

As each contraction starts, gently blow a breath out, letting go of any muscles which have started to tighten as you anticipate the contraction. Then take a slow breath in through your nose and try to get that ball of air down from the top half of your chest to the bottom of your lungs. Next breathe the air out through your mouth with a gentle puff. Thereafter breathe in and out as deeply as is comfortable, always thinking about relaxing on the outward breath. Finally, at the end of the contraction, breathe out a long sigh of relief – it will help relax all those muscles.

In between contractions aim to let go, and, if need be, stretch any remaining tension out of your muscles as you would in a relaxation session. If you can keep the tension in the muscles to a minimum, you will find you cope much better with each contraction as it comes and have a clear head for any decisions you need to make. It is helpful if your partner reminds you at the beginning of each contraction to breathe out as calmly as you can.

Never mind if the breathing technique sometimes goes wrong during a contraction. Just start again with the next. If at any point you get into a panic and begin gasping or overbreathing, you may find it easier to restore the pattern either by a loud exclamation to release tension or by repeating a series of little outward breaths, such as 'Ha Ha Hoooo' or 'Sh Sh Shhhh'. Your partner can help you with this by patting out the rhythm on your hand. And cursing or groaning – simply letting everyone know how you feel – not only releases emotional tension but also makes you breathe out slowly, so helping to re-establish a regular pattern of breathing.

When it comes to the second, pushing stage of labour, whether you find it easier to hold your breath or let it out as you bear down is up to you. You may have heard famous tennis players letting out a grunting breath as they put all their energies into a shot: the technique could help you too. If you can make two or three bearing-down actions during each pushing contraction rather than one long one, you will be less likely to exhaust yourself and the baby. If you have difficulty getting the hang of pushing, blow on your fist as on page 81 and feel your diaphragm pushing down on your bump and your pelvic floor bulging out. It is this action you are aiming for every time you push. You can do this when you are practising to find a comfortable birth position.

After the birth
In the days after the baby is born, breathing and relaxation techniques can help you cope with 'afterpains' as your uterus gradually contracts to its normal size (you may not experience these with a first baby) or with soreness following a Caesarean.

Relaxation can also be a great help with breastfeeding, particularly if you are a little unsure at the beginning. And establishing a breastfeeding ritual will help to make feeds go more easily. If you have a chair you always feed in plus a bag with everything you are likely to need – spare nappies, cotton wool, tissues, creams and spare clothing – you will save last-minute rushing about and you will find that your body soon learns to 'think' milk. Instead of needing to relax to feed, it will have learned to relax you *by* feeding.

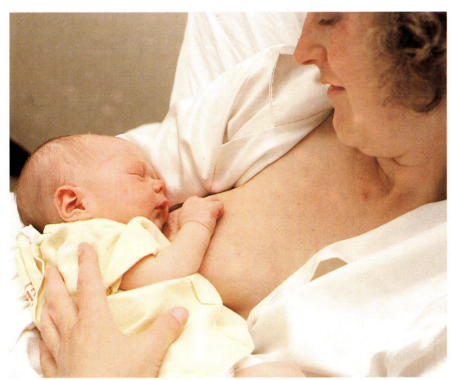

≈ MASSAGE ≈

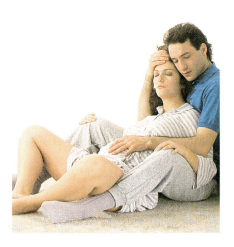

*O*ne of the best and most effective ways of deepening an understanding between yourself and someone who is special to you is through massage. Massage can vary from a smooth caress to the firm rubbing of a bruised muscle. Its important physiological effects on the body have been demonstrated scientifically. It is known to relax tense muscles, to improve blood pressure and to reduce pain. It benefits both the person who is stroked and the person doing the stroking as anyone who owns a cat or dog will be aware.

Massage is an excellent way of really getting to know the feel of your body and that's important during pregnancy. If you and your partner can explore your changing shape from the earliest stages of pregnancy, not only will you cope better during labour and breastfeeding because you are more in tune with your body, but you should both enjoy greater physical and emotional closeness.

Massage can also add a pleasurable extra to lovemaking at any time: it can be particularly useful towards the end of pregnancy when full intercourse is sometimes uncomfortable. And after the birth it is an excellent aid to relaxation, when tiredness and disorientation can make it difficult to find the time and desire for sex at first.

Massage has a place in labour too. An age-old response to pain has been to 'rub it better'. The pains and discomforts of labour tend to respond to rhythmical, gentle stroking, which can not only soothe and help make the pain more bearable but can do much to keep the breathing calm during contractions. Between contractions it can be a great aid to relaxation, particularly towards the end of the first stage of labour, when the intervals are considerably shorter. It can also be very calming to the nerves if you are waiting to have a Caesarean.

The key to successful massage is to stroke with confidence. You will gain that confidence with practice as both you and your partner discover the pleasure that can be given and received from it. But when you first begin practising massage or when trying out a new method, don't expect it to work brilliantly from the very beginning. You may need to discuss what you are doing and how it feels. You can demonstrate on your partner how you would like to be massaged if finding words is difficult. When done with tender care and consideration, massage is an unspoken language of sharing, understanding and encouragement.

Breaking down barriers
Although massage can be a deeply pleasurable experience, dispelling troubles and providing a real source of comfort when in pain, not everyone likes to be touched. If you or your partner feel this way and would like to ease the source of tension, then you will find it easiest if you think first of all about those parts of your body and those circumstances in which you least mind being touched. Even the most sensitive people have some ways of experiencing physical contact which they find acceptable. It may be letting somebody else wash their hair, scratch their back, sponge them with cold water when hot or simply holding hands. Start from there, become aware of how your body feels when it is touched on those occasions and find ways of making what is already a safe experience enjoyable. Once you are really enjoying it, gradually move on to new approaches. Take your time and, if you find one technique difficult, try something different.

'Doing massage has brought us together much more. It has provided a physical closeness which we had rather lost after the early months of being married.'

Basic techniques

Massage is best done on bare skin. If the skin is particularly sensitive, try wearing a thin cotton garment or use a little oil or talcum powder. Both you and your partner need to be in comfortable positions. The person being stroked must be well supported: this is particularly important in the case of head and neck massage, when unnecessary effort can be spent trying to keep the head in position. If standing to do the massage, this means having your feet hip width apart to distribute the weight equally and keeping your back straight. If kneeling or sitting, you should be able to stroke either away from your body or towards it.

1

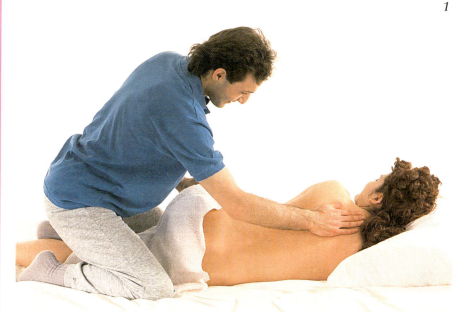

POSITIONS
□ *Kneel with one knee either side of the partner's body while he or she lies on one side (**1**) Uses: back, arm and thigh massage*
□ *Stand behind your partner as he or she sits on an upright chair. If the man is standing, a* cushion between his body and the back of his partner's neck may be necessary for support. Uses: head, neck and shoulder massage
□ *Kneel at chest level beside your partner who lies on his or her stomach with the head resting on the arms. Or stand* behind your partner as he or she sits astride an upright chair and leans forward over the back of it. Uses: neck massage
□ *Sit at right angles to each other with your partner's feet on your lap, the legs straight and slightly raised. Uses: foot and leg massage*

THE RIGHT PACE

Massage strokes should be firm, smooth and rhythmical. Sometimes the rhythm will be fairly quick, as when kneading or rubbing a sore place, but it should be slower when the intention is to soothe: for example, take about 5 seconds to stroke down the full length of the back. You should always aim to stroke the whole length of a part of the body. So, if you are stroking the thighs you should stroke from the hip along the thigh bone to the knee (2). Or, in the case of the back, from the nape of the neck down the full length of the spine to the tail bone. Stroking the full length is not only more satisfying but it helps prevent the pace speeding up.

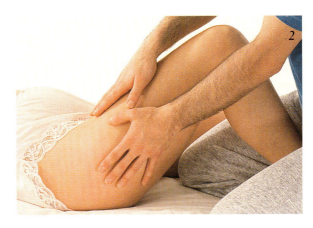

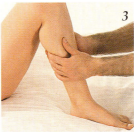

KNEADING AND STROKING

Kneading or squeezing (3) and releasing handfuls of muscle is good for cramps but follow with stroking to soothe, using the palm of the hand to avoid tickling.

CIRCULAR RUBBING

Applying pressure with the ball of the thumb, fingertips or the heel of the hand (4) can be a good way of providing relief for extremely tense muscles. Use a slow, even, circular motion. When massaging the small of the back, stand over your partner and rub with the heel of the hand so that the fingers point downwards.

COMMON FAULTS

Massaging too lightly will tickle and too fast will irritate. Pace and firmness depend on your preference, but the best way of showing your partner what you like is to demonstrate on him or her.

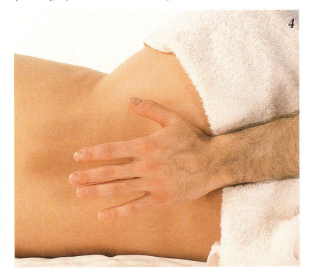

Massage for relaxation

*T*hese suggestions can be the basis for your own ideas. Anything which relaxes and soothes you both can be put to use.

BODY MASSAGE
Using the flat of the hand, rest your palm on the nape of your partner's neck and then stroke firmly and smoothly down the full length of the spine. When you reach the tail bone, place your hand once more on the nape of the neck and stroke again, remembering to slow down rather than speed up. You can do this using one hand over and over again or using both hands alternately (1).

This is also a useful massage for anyone who is having difficulty getting to sleep.

In the same way you can gently stroke other parts of the body, such as the tummy (2) or thighs.

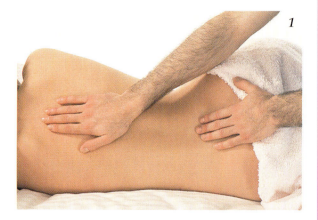

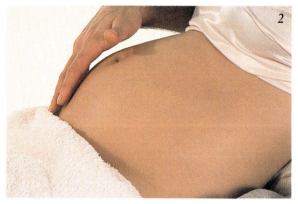

HEAD MASSAGE
There are two ways of stroking the forehead. Most people have a definite preference for one or the other.

Using the flat of your hands, stroke from the line of the eyebrows back to as near the crown of the head as possible (3). If you use both hands

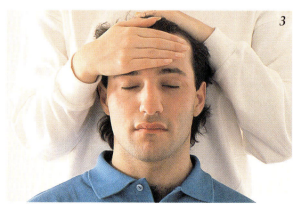

alternately, the stroking is almost continuous.

With the tips of your fingers facing each other and touching the brow directly above your partner's nose, smooth them away from each other along the brow (**4**) until just behind the ears and then repeat.
You can also apply gentle circular pressure to the temples and to the scalp as if washing the hair.

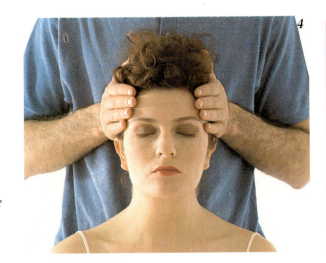

NECK AND
SHOULDER MASSAGE
The person receiving the massage should be seated astride a chair, leaning forward facing the back and supporting his or her chest with a cushion, or lying on his or her stomach.

Start by kneading the fleshy part of the shoulders near the base of the neck. Then apply gentle pressure with the fingers and thumbs at the base of the skull(**5**). Next apply circular pressure at the base of the neck on either side of the spine: get your partner to tell you which spot feels right. Finally, with the flat of your hands, stroke the upper arms (**6**) from the top of the shoulder or from the armpit to the elbow (depending on their position).

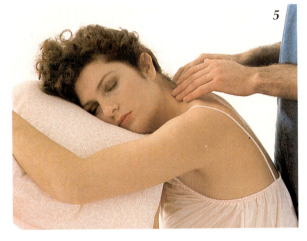

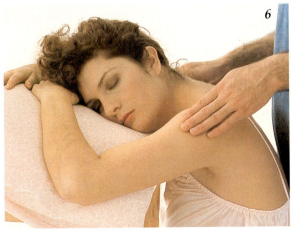

Intimate massage

Massage, unlike making love, has the advantage that it can be done virtually anywhere. It relaxes and soothes the tension that family life can bring, it encourages the physical closeness which both partners need and it is a wonderful way of saying 'I love you'.

Making time to give each other a 5- or 10-minute massage each day will be good for you both. It could be some head, neck and shoulder massage for your partner after a day's work, back stroking to encourage a good night's sleep, back and shoulder massage to ease backache, or leg massage after long periods of standing. Even if you start in a rather unwilling state of mind, you will soon find that the hypnotic effect of the rhythmical strokes takes over. The first massage described below is the kind of all-body massage you can both enjoy. Try it out or, even better, make up your own.

Whole-body sequence
Starting with the back, use the flat of both hands to stroke from the small of the back up on either side of the spine to the shoulders and then across them and down the sides to the bottom of the spine again. Repeat several times. If nervousness makes your partner ticklish, then stroke more firmly. Once he or she is truly relaxed, you can do more delicate stroking if you wish.

Next, massage downwards on both sides of the thigh nearest you until you reach the knee. Repeat several times, and then do the same from the knee down to the ankle. Stroke the sole of the foot several times. Gently push the foot so that the toes point up to stretch the back of the leg and ankle and repeat the foot stroking.

Let that foot rest in your hands for a few moments before you start on the other leg. Keeping your hands still for a short while on one part of the body before moving onto the next is warming and it signals gentleness and care. Abrupt movements in massage can be very jarring. So, when you finish the sequence, rest your hands on your partner's body and then remove them slowly and gently so as not to disrupt the sensation of peace and contentment.

Perineal massage
Insert a thumb into your vagina and gently stroke the base of it backwards and forwards in a U-shaped curve. Once you are accustomed to this technique, you can massage more vigorously and eventually use both thumbs. You should be able to feel your perineum beginning to stretch. Maintain that level of pressure for 30–60 seconds so that you can accustom yourself to the sensation and then relax the muscles. The more you can 'let go' of the perineal

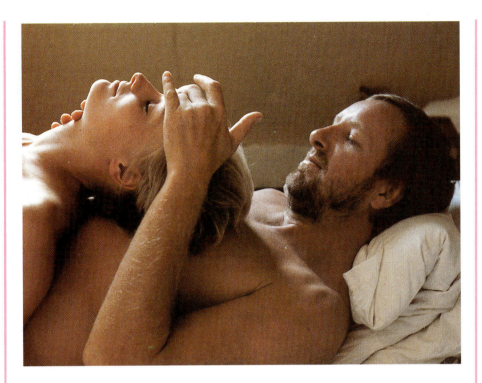

muscles, the easier it will be for them to 'give' during the birth. Some midwives believe perineal massage for six weeks before the birth and during labour reduces the need for an episiotomy – a surgical cut in the perineum – and subsequent stitches.

Breast massage
This helpful preparation for breastfeeding is one you can practise in the bath. Using the flat of the hands, place the heel of each hand either side of one breast and *gently* stroke towards the nipple. Next place one hand on top and the other underneath the breast and again stroke towards the nipple. Repeat for the other breast, making sure the whole of each breast is stroked. Then gently stretch the pigmented area around each nipple with your index fingers, sideways and from top to bottom. If the nipples are flat, this exercise will help them to stand out.

You may find you produce a few drops of colostrum: massaging the breasts in this way is the basis of the technique for expressing milk and can be useful if you suffer any tender swelling – engorgement – of the breasts as is possible in the early days of breastfeeding. Massaging the nipples by gently rolling them between thumb and index finger has also been shown to help stimulate contractions during labour.

Massage for labour

When you are in labour, massage can be very reassuring. Being able to *feel* the physical presence of your partner or someone who cares can often bring additional relief to the simple knowledge that that person is present. And the calmer and more confident the touch, the calmer and more confident you will both be.

Firm massage in early labour may become uncomfortable later on. A gently resting hand may be all that is wanted and, if even that feels unbearable, sponging with cold water, fanning to keep cool or simply your partner's voice may be the most welcome form of contact.

Between contractions, which last only 1–2 minutes, you and your partner can discuss what might help you. Partners can also experiment; changing methods prevents them from overtiring their own muscles. However, they should remember that the object of massage is to soothe and comfort, not to release their own tension. Short, hesitant touches will do neither of you any good, whereas establishing a steady, smooth rhythm will be calming for you both. If you have practised massage during your pregnancy, you will both know what 'feels' best and how to communicate if labour becomes difficult at any point.

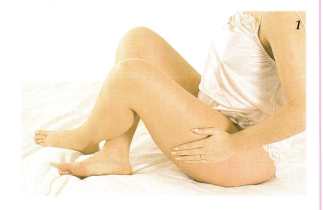

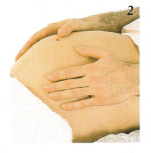

THIGH MASSAGE
Either kneel with your knees wide apart and sit back on your heels, maybe with a couple of books or pillows under your bottom for support, or sit cross-legged. Then, placing your hands on the outsides of your thighs, stroke down to the knee (1) and back up on the insides, across to your hips and round again. As you stroke forwards, you can swing your body forwards too, combining a rocking action with the stroking movement. This is good for contractions felt in the thighs or tummy.

TUMMY MASSAGE
Using the fingertips, do a figure-of-eight movement across the body under the bump (2). Keep the touch light if the tummy is very painful. Good for contractions felt like period pains.

BACK MASSAGE

Apply circular pressure to the small of the back with the heel of the hand (**3**), or hold alternately a hot-water bottle and an ice pack (as used in a picnic box) against the small of the back. Both are good for contractions felt in the back. See also back stroking on page 102.

Back-pressure massage can be hard work and you can get equally good relief using the pressure of a rolling pin. You should lean forwards, supported by cushions, over the back of a chair so that your back is straight or slightly hollowed. Your partner should be behind you, kneeling with one knee raised. He places the rolling pin on the small of your back, or wherever comfortable, and then, using his body weight, rocks back and forth so that the rolling pin rolls up and down about 7.5–10cm (3–4in) above and below the small of the back.

You can use a rolling pin yourself to ease back ache by positioning it between the small of your back and a door frame and then bending and straightening the knees a few inches to achieve the same effect.

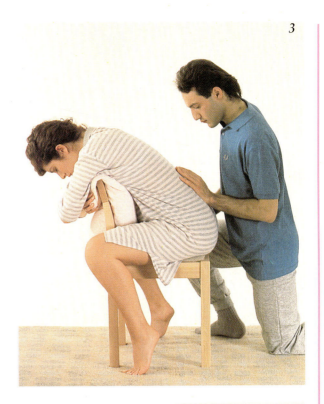

HAND MASSAGE

One of the simplest and easiest contacts is simply to hold, pat or stroke a hand (**4**). If you want to hold hands during labour, the important thing is for your partner to hold your hand, not the other way round. Then you can relax into the touch.

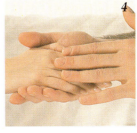

FACE MASSAGE

A small sponge dipped in cold water, wrung out and smoothed over the forehead, down the sides of the cheeks and the nose and across the chin can be comforting.

IN THE BATH

Kneeling in a deep warm bath can be soothing and your partner can set up a helpful rhythm by pouring cups of warm water over your back. Being washed with a damp flannel and dried with a towel can be welcome if labour is making you uncomfortable.

Massage for babies

New mothers have a particularly heightened awareness in the early days after birth which makes them feel the need to get to know as much about their babies as they are able. It is this increased sensitivity that can also make you so emotional at first – naturally overwhelmed by the wonder of it all. The more your baby is with you, the more use you can make of this natural response by simply looking, touching and listening. You may never have found other babies fascinating, but if you allow yourself to touch and get to know your own baby well, you will soon find yourself coming under her spell. Simply stroking and enjoying your baby's soft skin, little movements and noises will make you feel protective and help physical and emotional closeness to grow.

WHOLE-BODY MASSAGE

Just before or just after a bath, when your baby is undressed, is a good time to practise, provided she is not too hungry. Lie her on her tummy and lightly stroke from her shoulders to her feet several times (1) and then from her shoulders to her fingertips. Turn her over onto her back and stroke the front of her body.

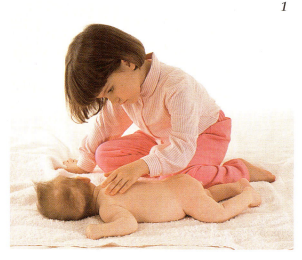

1

FACE MASSAGE

Lie the baby on your lap facing you and, using your fingertips, stroke her forehead, from the middle outwards (2). Using your thumbs, stroke the tops of her cheeks and then, with your fingertips, stroke the sides of her face to meet at her chin.

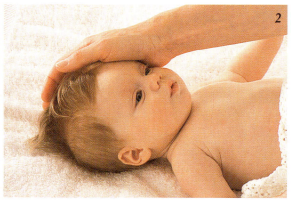

2

You will inevitably touch your baby frequently as you attend to her needs, but this is not the same as taking the time to touch for the sheer pleasure of it. Massaging, like feeding, involves rhythms which nappy changing, dressing and undressing do not. Giving your baby a massage is soothing for both of you and allows an opportunity to enjoy the feel of each other. You can begin as soon as she starts to have periods of wakefulness. Use light but firm pressure, taking your guide from how she reacts. Being able to stroke your child confidently will be a useful technique throughout childhood.

Your toddler will want to touch the new baby too and can be shown ways of stroking her or simply feeling her softness and noticing her dimples. This will encourage the older child to feel protective as well as giving satisfaction because he can soothe the newcomer. It's safer, of course, to let him practise stroking while the baby is lying down, rather than while holding her.

FOOT AND HAND MASSAGE

'This little piggy' can be an opportunity gently to stretch her toes (3) and uncurl her fingers. Simply sitting your baby on your lap and stroking her hands and feet with your thumbs will help keep her contented and it's something you can do even when visitors claim your attention.

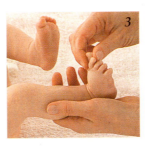

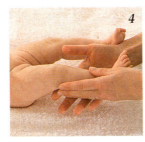

ARM AND LEG MASSAGE

Lie the baby on her back and, lifting her legs, either do bicycling movements or gently stroke her legs (4) letting her push against your hands with her feet. You can also do large circular movements with her arms. All help the baby enjoy the feel of muscles being gently stretched.

TUMMY MASSAGE

Stroking with gentle, even pressure on a baby's tummy can help soothe colic. Either lie her over your knees with her bottom slightly higher than her head and pat her bottom (firmly if there is a good padding of nappy) or stroke the sides of her tummy from the hips up to the chest. Or lie her on her back and circle her tummy button (5) with both hands stroking in the same direction.

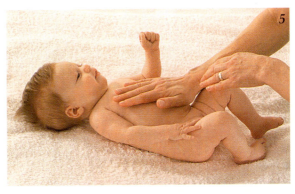

THE MEDICAL BACKGROUND

Understanding your antenatal care, the medical terms you will come across and the amazing development of your growing baby can help you to feel more confident throughout your pregnancy and labour.

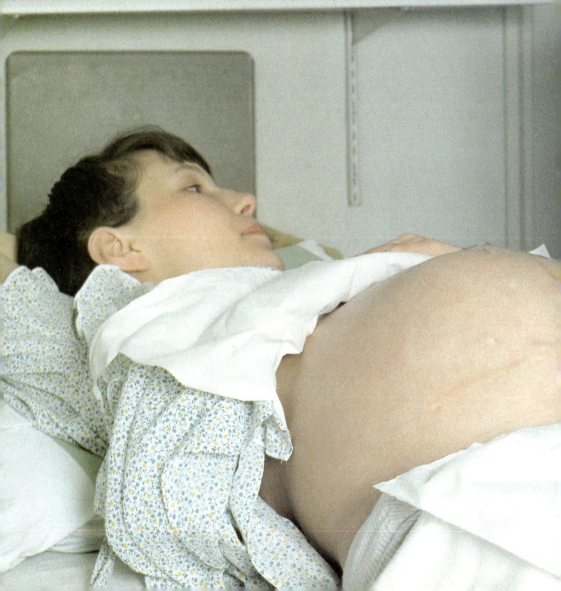

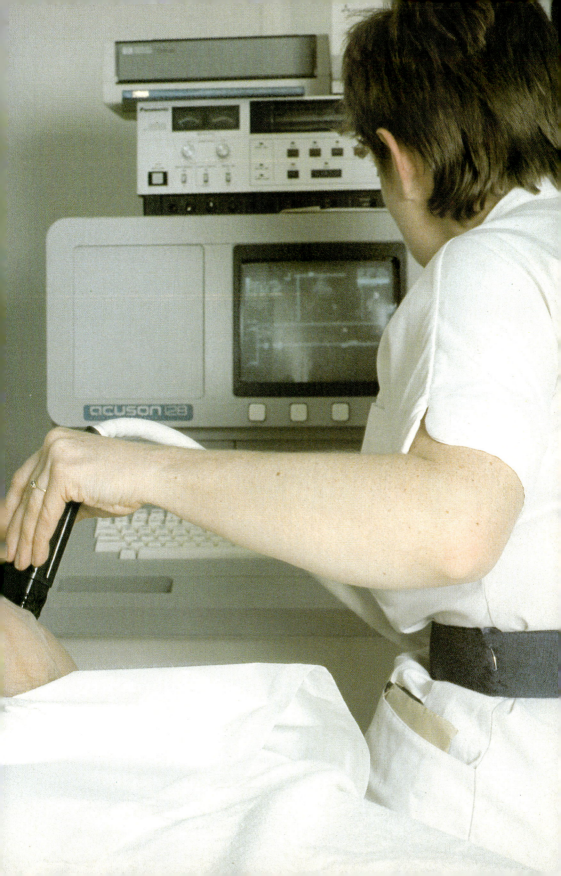

Your medical care

*B*elow is your likely programme of medical care during pregnancy and after, if you are expecting your first baby. If you have had a baby before, everything was straightforward and there are no complications this time, you may have fewer check-ups: ask your doctor or midwife what to expect.

6–8 weeks
Visit your GP for confirmation that you are pregnant and to discuss where you will have your baby. Not all options listed below may be available in your area. Ask your doctor about any which interest you. He or she may mention only those which suit him or her.

Full hospital care All your antenatal check-ups and the birth take place in hospital. If there is more than one hospital in your area, find out which might suit you best. The same goes for your consultant. Although you may never see him, he can have a marked influence on the type of care you receive, depending on whether he is more or less 'technologically' minded. Your GP will probably recommend the one he or she gets on with best.

Shared care Your antenatal care is divided between a GP and the hospital. If your GP does not provide antenatal care, you can ask for a temporary referral for your maternity care. Ask around to find a GP you can expect to like. You can still go to your own doctor for any other care. You may need to choose your hospital and consultant.

GP unit care Some hospitals have a unit where GPs who belong to the scheme can deliver their patients' babies. Antenatal care is handled by the GP or midwife and one or other delivers you in the special unit.

Domino scheme 'Domino' is short for domiciliary in-and-out scheme, in which a midwife is mainly responsible for your antenatal care. She comes to your home when labour begins, goes with you to hospital and returns home with you six hours after birth as long as there are no complications.

Home birth Your GP may not be prepared to do this but, provided there are no medical reasons why a home birth is not advisable, he or she can refer you to a GP who is willing. If you cannot find a GP, write to the Director of Midwifery Services at your local hospital; she is legally obliged to provide you with a midwife.

Once you have selected your option, your doctor will make the necessary arrangements and give you information about free prescriptions and dental treatment. If you are not happy with the scheme you choose, find out about the alternatives and discuss with your GP or midwife the possibility of changing.

10–12 weeks
Your first visit to the hospital antenatal clinic for booking in. A midwife will take down your medical history and you can discuss pregnancy care and where to go for antenatal classes. A doctor will give you a general examination, including blood pressure, urine and weight, plus blood tests to determine blood group, haemoglobin level and any diseases which can be detected in this way. This tends to be a long visit.

16 weeks
You will have an alpha-fetoprotein blood test to check for certain problems in the baby, such as spina bifida, and an ultrasound scan at the hospital to confirm that the baby is the correct size for your dates.

Second antenatal check-up: your weight, urine, blood pressure, whether you have oedema and height of the uterus will be checked from now on.

20 weeks
Third antenatal check-up. You will be asked if you can feel your baby moving yet.

24 weeks
Fourth antenatal check-up: the fetal heart will be listened for from now on – unless the baby is obviously kicking.

28 weeks
Fifth antenatal check-up. If you are under shared care, it will be a long session at the hospital. Your haemoglobin level will be checked. You will get a certificate of expected confinement and be told how to claim maternity benefit. You should know by now when your antenatal classes start.

30 weeks
Sixth antenatal check-up.

32 weeks
Seventh antenatal check-up.

34 weeks
Eighth antenatal check-up. If having shared care, this will be at hospital, perhaps with the consultant, and may include a blood test. The baby's position will be noted from now on.

36 weeks
Ninth antenatal check-up.

37 weeks and weekly until birth
Tenth antenatal check-up and so on, usually at the hospital now if having shared care.

After the birth
Paediatrician will check the baby on the day of birth and before you go home a few days later. While you are in hospital, a midwife will check your health daily, a physiotherapist will advise you on exercise and a family-planning nurse will discuss contraception. At home, a community midwife will visit you daily until the tenth day or longer, if necessary.

10th day after birth
Health visitor will visit, telling you about clinics and how often she will call at your home.

6 weeks
Postnatal check-up for you with your GP or in hospital, including possibly a cervical smear test and family-planning discussion. Developmental check for your baby by a paediatrician or child-health specialist.

Your progress through pregnancy

0–12 weeks

THE BABY By 12 weeks the baby is recognizably human, though it is only about 6.5cm (2½in) long and weighing less than 25g (1oz). The heart, liver and lungs are all distinguishable and beginning to work but they have yet to be refined. The baby is already quite active, though curled up, and can swallow the surrounding amniotic fluid as well as being able to bend knees, elbows and wrists. These movements are too tiny to be felt. The eyes are closed and it is not yet possible to see if the baby is a boy or a girl.

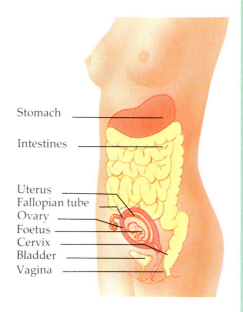

Stomach

Intestines

Uterus
Fallopian tube
Ovary
Foetus
Cervix
Bladder
Vagina

YOU Your breasts have grown and may feel tender and tingly. The areola around the nipple may have darkened and you can see some raised bumps there. You may feel sick and be extremely tired. Hormonal changes and pressure from the uterus, which is getting bigger inside the pelvis, may make you want to empty your bladder frequently. The placenta, a flat, spongy organ like the liver, is taking shape. The development of a healthy placenta is more important to your baby's wellbeing than your physical health.

16 weeks

THE BABY The baby is about 15cm (6in) long and weighs about 150g (5oz). The sex is now easily identified. Nails have formed on her fingers and toes, and downy hair is beginning to grow all over her body. Her movements feel like a gentle fluttering or bubbling sensation, though if this is your first baby you may have difficulty recognizing them for another few weeks. She can suck her fingers

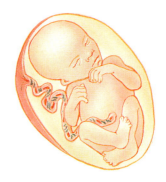

and pass out through her kidneys and bladder the fluid she is swallowing. Her heart is beating very fast, about 140 times a minute, so that the equivalent of about 28 litres (50 pints) of blood a day circulate between it and the placenta. The ultrasound scan taken about now will look very blurry or quite clear, depending on how your baby is lying, but the shape and internal organs are identifiable to the trained eye. From now on the baby is growing in size, the muscles are developing though she is very skinny, a layer of grease, called vernix, covers her body to protect the skin from becoming waterlogged and she becomes more active so you soon feel definite movement.

YOU Any sickness or tiredness should begin to ease off as you enter this stage of pregnancy. Hormones are softening your ligaments as well as other body tissues in preparation for the birth, and constipation may be one consequence. You may notice changes in your skin and hair. A dark line of pigment, the *linea nigra*, may appear, running between your tummy button and your pubic hair. From now on your bump continues to grow out and to rise higher in the abdomen so that you cannot button up a skirt. You feel too big for your ordinary clothes but are swamped by maternity clothes.

28 weeks

THE BABY She is 35.5cm (14in) long and weighs about 900g (2lb). She is extremely thin, having almost no body fat. Her grip is now probably at its most powerful and she could support her own body weight by hanging on. She has the waste product meconium in her bowels. If your doctor/midwife suggests it, you may be able to hear her heart beat through a monitor or stethoscope. If your baby were born now, she would have a high chance of survival under intensive care. The eyelids open for the first time.

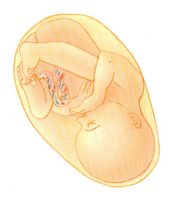

YOU Heartburn, leg cramps and breathlessness may be a problem. Drops of colostrum may be secreted from the nipples. Giving up work any time now, antenatal classes and increased awareness of the baby's presence may make you think more about birth.

32 weeks
THE BABY She is about 40cm (16in) long and weighs about 1.6kg (3½lb). The internal surfaces of the lungs are beginning to develop little bubbles of surfactant, which prevent the newborn baby's lungs from collapsing so that she is able to breathe on her own. This lung development can be checked, if necessary. She is beginning to receive antibodies from you which can protect her from infections and she is starting to put on fat. The bones are rapidly storing up calcium so that they harden, and stores of other minerals and vitamins are beginning to build up. She can suck but, if born now, she would have difficulty coordinating her breathing and swallowing actions, which is why she would need to receive most of her food by tube. From now on she should start to settle into a head-down position. You may be aware when the baby has hiccups or 'jumps' if startled by a sudden, loud noise. A pattern of sleeping and waking is taking shape, and when she is awake she can seem to leap, wriggle, bounce, twist and turn.

YOU From now on you will become steadily heavier and look more and more pregnant. You may be aware of contractions during which your bump rises to a peak along the *linea nigra*. These contractions may vary from quite painful to totally painless. You will also be able to see moving lumps on your abdomen as the baby turns over or moves her fists and feet; stabbing 'indigestion' may be the baby kicking your stomach. Stretch marks may appear and you may feel hot and sweat more. If your baby were born now, your breasts would produce milk of a rich composition suited to her extra needs.

36 weeks
THE BABY She is filling out and gaining about 225g (8oz) in weight each week. There is less amniotic fluid as the baby takes up more and more space and her movements may begin to slow down as she has less room. Rubbing against the walls of the uterus also causes the downy body hair and vernix covering to wear off gradually. If this is your first baby, her head may have 'engaged', or slipped down snugly into the pelvis, but do not assume that this is an indication of early labour.

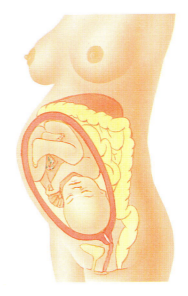

YOU The uterus is now about the highest it will get and it may be pressing on your lungs and stomach, making eating large meals and breathing difficult. Sleeping may be a problem too. Once the baby's head drops down, your bladder may be squashed so that you feel the need to empty your bladder more frequently but without actually producing much urine. Your pelvic bones are now extremely flexible, your vulva may be greatly enlarged and your vagina may be almost purple in colour. From now on the birth may be imminent so you should collect all the things you will need for labour. Waiting may make you impatient and fed up with pregnancy discomforts.

Birth and after

THE BABY She is about 50cm (20in) in length and the skull bones are still soft enough to be squeezed lengthways as the head passes down the birth canal. She has enough fat to stop her body temperature from dropping too rapidly and to prevent her being hungry for the first couple of days as she adjusts to sucking. Stores of other nutrients, like iron, will last her the first few months of life. The antibodies she had begun to receive from your blood will continue to be supplied through your colostrum and breast milk until her body is able to make her own. The liver is still not fully mature, which is why a baby may have difficulty eliminating drugs like pethidine,

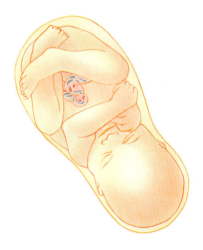

sometimes offered in labour. The kidneys also have still to mature. For this reason babies need special baby-milk formulas if they are not breastfed and should not be fed salt in weaning foods for the first year.

YOU The onset of labour may be heralded by a spurt of unexpected activity, a small loss in weight and loose bowels. The mucous plug in the neck of the womb may come away with some blood as a 'show' at the onset of labour or several days before. The baby's head engages at the onset of labour, if it has not already done so. The contractions which increase and intensify during labour and birth decline and are felt as 'afterpains' as the uterus contracts to its prepregnant size. The hormones produced in labour trigger off the production of colostrum and later breast milk. As your baby gets older, the composition of your milk changes to match her changing needs.

Common complaints in pregnancy and childbirth

Aching legs
Exercise using the warm-up routines for legs, feet and ankles on page 76. If your legs often ache, do these exercises frequently to stimulate the circulation and stretch the muscles.

Anaemia
This condition occurs when the blood is deficient in either red colouring, haemoglobin, or red-blood cells so that insufficient oxygen is transferred from the blood to the tissues. The normal haemoglobin level is 12–13 grams per 100 ml but it appears lower in pregnancy because the blood is diluted with extra fluid. If the level drops below 10 ½ grams a woman may be prescribed iron and folate tablets to prevent serious shortage.

Baby in awkward position
Some midwives believe that babies who are lying in awkward positions – for example, on their backs against the mother's spine (posterior position) – can be encouraged to turn and get into the comfortable side-facing position if the mother gets on all fours for 10 minutes a day in the last six weeks of pregnancy.

Alternatively, you can rest, lying forward on a bean bag.

Backache
Either sit well back in a chair so that your back is straight or use the sitting position described on page 65. The latter takes the weight of the bump away from your back, and the weight of your body is supported both at the top and bottom of the trunk. Your partner can also massage your back in this position (see page 107). Alternatively, lie on your back with your legs straight, bend one knee and take that foot over the other leg, tucking it under the other knee; then slowly curve the whole of your back over to stretch the spine. Repeat, using the other leg. The squat and pelvic tilt (see pages 78 and 80) can also relieve pain in the lower back.

Blood-pressure changes
If your blood pressure suddenly rises or if the lower reading (diastolic pressure) reaches 90, you may be advised to rest more. However, if resting in bed simply makes you more tense and restless, you are unlikely to receive much benefit. Practise the relaxation exercise on page 93 and try to get away from any source of

anxiety. Taking a woman into hospital can sometimes help because her other duties have to be delegated. Low blood-pressure is common in pregnancy and is harmless.

Breathlessness
A need to breathe more deeply is common in pregnancy but it can be made difficult if the baby is pressing on your lungs or if you constantly slouch, preventing the air from reaching the bottom of your lungs. Try leaning forwards over the back of a chair (see page 65) and learning the deep-breathing technique on page 94 will also help stop breathlessness and any subsequent agitation.

Clumsiness
The hormone progesterone causes fluid retention and softening of the ligaments around the joints, sometimes making it difficult to have full control over your limbs so it can be easy for your ankle to give way suddenly or for you to find yourself dropping things. Falls are also more common. None of these incidents is likely to cause the baby any harm. They are simply annoying and

you will need to take extra care of yourself.

Constipation

The pregnancy hormones can cause the intestines to become sluggish: confirmation that your body is relaxing and opening up in preparation for the birth. See page 49 for treatment. Opening your bowels can also provide an opportunity for practising bearing-down exercises for the birth (see page 81).

Faintness or dizziness

This is most common in the early weeks of pregnancy and is caused by a slowing down of the circulation and a subsequent drop in blood pressure. As the blood supply increases, feelings of faintness disappear. Avoid getting up suddenly or standing for long periods. Take things slowly and sit down as much as possible, putting your head between your knees if you begin to feel light-headed.

Fluid retention or oedema

Arms and legs which are a little puffy due to extra fluid are not a sign of ill-health on their own, but the condition can be extremely uncomfortable nonetheless. Puffiness of the eyes or face should always be reported to your doctor or midwife. Vigorous foot exercises, including pumping the feet up and down at least 30 times regularly throughout the day (see page 76) and keeping the feet raised whenever possible, will also help swollen ankles and feet. Ice packs on the affected area may help too.

Hair loss

This is more apparent than real after the baby is born (see page 24). It is not a sign that you are going bald.

Headache

If this happens in early pregnancy, your doctor may suggest an eye test. Otherwise ease the muscular tension at the back of the head with neck and shoulder exercises (see page 77) or massage (see page 102). If headaches are frequent or severe, contact your doctor.

Heartburn and indigestion

See page 48 for an explanation and for treatment. Some people also find resting after a meal helps, others prefer exercise, such as walking.

Itchiness of skin

See page 26 for treatment. Don't stay in the bath too long because soaking will remove even more of the skin's natural moisturizers. Moisturizing creams and oils rubbed into the skin may also help.

Leaking of urine

This is most common when you cough, sneeze or laugh and can occur at the beginning and end of pregnancy, when the uterus may be pressing down on the bladder, and after the birth when the muscles have been stretched. If it is bad enough to need a sanitary towel, take more general exercise and practise tightening the pelvic floor (see page 81).

Leg cramps

No one knows the cause but they can be triggered if the toes are pointed after the legs have been still for a time. During an attack of cramp, stretch the back of the legs with the heels pushed down and the toes pulled up. After bad cramps give the calf muscles a vigorous massage to prevent the subsequent ache (see page 101).

Nausea and sickness

This can be morning, evening or all-day sickness and is particularly common in the first three months of pregnancy. See page 48 for explanation and treatment.

Nightmares and vivid dreams

These are most common in the last three months of pregnancy. Everyone dreams several times a night but remembers very little; because sleep difficulties are more common towards the end of pregnancy it is easier for pregnant women to remember dreams. They are not a sign that something is wrong with either your baby or you. However, it is quite natural to be anxious that everything will be all right after the baby is born and this may manifest itself in strange dreams, even if you are not consciously worrying during the day.

Nose bleeds and stuffy nose

Both conditions are due to hormonal changes which affect the lining of the nose so treat it gently. If a nose bleed is profuse and prolonged, see your doctor. Hold the nose for about 10 minutes if bleeding is bad, to let a clot form.

Pain below the bump

A dull ache or sharp dragging pain below the bump is caused by the softening of the ligaments. It more often occurs on the left than the right side and can be eased with the support of a maternity girdle or simply by propping up your bump from underneath with your hands. If you need to cough or laugh, try to bend your knees to avoid a sharp pull on the ligaments. See also page 65 for advice on how to get up from a lying position.

Pain between the shoulders

This is probably caused by softened ligaments and bad posture. See page 77 for exercise and page 103 for massage.

Pain in the buttocks or thighs

The loosening of the pelvic joints and softening of the ligaments in the sacroiliac area (just below the dimples at the base of the spine) can cause aching and a feeling of stiffness after sitting and lying down. See page 64 for comfortable sitting position. Clenching and releasing the buttocks may also help.

When you want to get up, shift your weight to the front of the chair and then rock your pelvis backwards and forwards to ease the stiffness before rising. If you find it difficult to turn over in bed, draw your knees up and, keeping them together, roll onto your side.

If the pain is extremely bad, you may need the help of an obstetric physiotherapist – ask at the hospital.

Pain or tingling in the wrists or hands

This is caused by excess fluid pressing on the ligaments and nerves. Shake your hands and wrists frequently with your arms stretched above your head. Ice packs may help and, if the pain is really bad, you should ask to see an obstetric physiotherapist.

Piles or haemorrhoids

Be encouraged: they are a sign that you are softening up beautifully!

You can gently push the haemorrhoids back inside your anus with your finger when in the bath. They will stay with you until the birth. Massaging with an ice cube may numb pain and ease swelling. They can also be caused by pushing too early and for too long at birth.

Pressure in the vaginal area

This can happen if the baby's head engages before labour so that the circulation becomes congested in this area. Lying down so that the baby's head falls back a little from the pelvis and squatting can help (see page 78).

Pubic pain

The ligaments may soften so much that the pubic bones separate. Keeping still with your legs apart, using a couple of walking sticks and wearing a maternity girdle can help. This painful condition should be treated by an obstetric physiotherapist.

Ravenous hunger

You may experience severe hunger pangs during pregnancy and, provided you don't use this as an excuse to indulge in chocolate bars at the expense of healthier foods, it need not be a problem. If you are hungry and were not overweight before pregnancy, then eat more. See page 51 for suggestions for snacks.

Restless legs
A creeping sensation down the legs which is relieved by movement, the condition is usually brought on by tiredness so extra rest will help. It usually disappears after the birth.

Ribcage pain
If the baby's head is pressing on the ribcage making it very sore, raise the arm on the affected side above your head, bend it and, grasping the elbow with your other hand, pull sideways. The action lifts the ribcage up and out.

Sleeplessness
This is most common in the last few weeks of pregnancy. See page 30 for treatment.

Swollen ankles
Rest your feet on a stool and every 30 minutes do vigorous foot exercises to stimulate the circulation (see page 76). Support tights or stockings may also help.

Tiredness
This can be particularly draining at the beginning of pregnancy, when life can become a cycle of work, sleep and nothing else. It is probably made worse by the fact that you do not look pregnant so others do not make allowances for you. The tiredness will pass, though towards the end of pregnancy some women begin to feel very tired again.
    Take sandwiches to work so that you can fit a short nap into your lunch hour. Learn to ask people to give up their seats on buses – it may be easier to explain to a woman than a man that you are newly pregnant and need to sit down.
    If you have a toddler who does not take much rest, you may need to ask friends to have him for a couple of hours each day. This is a useful way of building up a mutual support group: mothers of young children will probably be pleased to be asked because it means they will find it easier to ask you if they are unwell or need a helping hand. You should also go to bed for a couple of hours as soon as your toddler has gone to bed in the evening.

Too much saliva
A common condition at the beginning of pregnancy, it may help to find someone else who has had the same problem so you don't feel so unusual.

Vaginal discharge
This is always increased in pregnancy and, provided it does not look or smell any different or cause any soreness, it does not matter. Wear cotton underwear and, if necessary, change your pants twice a day or use stick-on pantie liners. During pregnancy the colour of the vagina changes from pale pink to purple.

Varicose veins
Varicose veins in the leg can be eased by walking, wearing support stockings or tights and keeping the feet raised rather than down. Support tights should ideally be put on in bed first thing in the morning before the blood has had a chance to collect in the slack parts of the veins.
    More troublesome are those in the vulva as they feel so peculiar and can be very painful. Lying down eases the discomfort. However, they will not hamper the ' birth and disappear as the perineum stretches and smoothes out.

Weight gain
See page 43 for explanation. If you find you are eating for the sake of it, take more exercise as this may help adjust your appetite. Your figure will be best looked after if you concentrate on improving your muscle tone and general fitness. Slimming, if you need to, should be either done before pregnancy or after breastfeeding has finished.

Wind
The effect of progesterone on the intestines often makes wind (or flatus) a problem, particularly in the early part of pregnancy. Frequent relief in private will help by preventing the build-up of painful discomfort.

Glossary

Active birth
A mother takes the initiative in labour rather than expecting that the medical staff will take charge. It also often means moving about during labour.

Amniocentesis (1)
A procedure in which a small sample of the fluid surrounding the baby is drawn off and tested for certain abnormalities, such as genetic disorders. It creates a small risk of miscarriage in early pregnancy. It may also be done in later pregnancy in, for example, premature labour, to check the maturity of the baby.

Analgesic
A pain-relieving substance. In labour the three principal analgesic drugs are an epidural or pethidine, both administered by injection, and entonox (gas and oxygen), which is inhaled.

Anterior position
A term used to describe the baby facing the mother's back, the position adopted by most babies before labour starts.

Antibodies
A variety of proteins with different, characteristic shapes present in the white-blood cells. They fight infection by attaching themselves to 'foreign' proteins, such as those in germs, whose shape they complement – as in a jigsaw puzzle – so inactivating them.

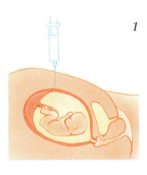

1

Artificial rupture of the membranes (ARM) or amniotomy
The piercing of the sac of membranes surrounding the baby with a surgical instrument. The membranes normally break of their own accord. Breaking them artificially to release the waters is done to speed up labour or to attach a fetal heart monitor. Contractions can be quicker and more painful after the waters break.

Assisted delivery
A baby has to be helped out of the woman's body by means of forceps or similar aid.

Braxton-Hicks contractions
The contractions of pregnancy, which may be felt occasionally from the beginning or not until the onset of labour.

Breech
A term used to describe the baby's position when it is bottom-downwards. A few babies are born bottom first.

Caesarean
The baby is delivered surgically by means of a cut through the abdominal wall, the mother being either asleep (under general anaesthetic) or awake (with an epidural).

Cephalic
A term used to describe the baby when it is head-downwards. The abbreviation 'C' or 'ceph' may be used on your medical notes.

Cervix
The neck of the uterus, plugged with thick mucus during pregnancy. Contractions in the first stage of labour narrow and draw up the cervix to make an opening for the baby from the uterus.

Coccyx
The tail bone at the base of the spine. Provided the woman is not sitting on it, it can move back during labour by as much as a quarter to create more space for the baby to be born.

Colostrum
Yellowish fluid produced by the breast which is rich in nutrients and antibodies and is the baby's first food for two or three days after birth.

Contractions
The muscular squeezing and stretching of the uterus felt during pregnancy and labour. During pregnancy contractions exercise the muscle wall of the uterus, enabling it to grow. Contractions last 1–2 minutes during labour.

Domino
The nickname for the 'domiciliary in-out' scheme, in which a mother is looked after by a community midwife, who comes to her home antenatally, accompanies her to hospital for the birth and back home a few hours later.

EDD (Expected day of delivery)
This is calculated as 40 weeks from the first day of the last period. It is only a rough guide. Most babies are born anytime between 37 and 43 weeks of pregnancy.

Enema
Purgatives are inserted into the bowel, usually as a pessary, to stimulate a bowel action. They are now much less common in childbirth because they neither reduce infection to the baby nor prevent soiling. They may be used if the woman is constipated or, occasionally, to trigger labour. If the bowels feel full during labour, it is because the baby's head is pressing on the rectum, not because the woman needs a bedpan.

Engorgement
Two or three days after the birth the breasts become bigger than ever, feeling hard, full and uncomfortable. This temporary condition is caused by an increase in normal body fluids as milk takes over from colostrum. It may also happen in the first two or three months if there is a longer gap than usual between feeds.

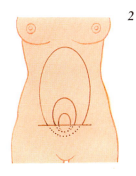

2

Entonox
An analgesic drug, composed of nitrous gas and oxygen, which may be breathed in through a mask or mouthpiece. Four or five deep inward breaths take about 20 seconds to work so it must be administered at the start of a contraction to be effective. It can be a useful short-term analgesic at the end of the first stage of labour, when the baby's head is crowning, or during stitching.

Epidural
A local anaesthetic which is injected into the lower spine to lessen the pain of labour contractions or to numb completely the lower half of the body for a Caesarean.

Episiotomy
A cut with a surgical instrument into the skin around the vagina to widen the birth opening, now usually performed only when there are birth difficulties. A local anaesthetic should be given first, but if the cut is made at the height of a contraction the pain will be no more than momentary at most.

Fetal-heart monitor
An electronic machine which gives a continuous record of the baby's heartbeat, usually by means of an electrode attached to his scalp or microphones taped to the mother's abdomen.

Fundus (2)
The upper part of the uterus. Its progressive height is checked from the second antenatal visit.

Haemorrhoids
Swollen varicose veins around the mouth of the anus, also known as piles.

Hypertension
High blood-pressure.

Induction
The artificial starting of labour by means of a vaginal pessary, a hormone drip into a vein or rupture of the sac of membranes.

Ligament
A strong band or sheet of fibrous tissue which either binds together bones or helps support internal organs such as the uterus.

LMP
Last menstrual period.

Meconium
The black, sticky waste contents of the fetus's bowels, normally excreted within two days after birth.

Mucus plug (3)
The protective plug of mucus at the neck of the uterus comes away during labour or a few days before, sometimes with a show of blood.

Natural birth
A rather unhelpful term which is usually taken to mean a birth that is 'drug-free' and with little medical intervention. Probably more important is a labour where the woman feels she is an equal member, or even the leader, of the team helping her give birth. Such births may or may not include the use of drugs and/or medical assistance.

Oxytocin
A hormone which stimulates labour

contractions and the production of milk.

Perineum
The area between the anus and the vagina.

Pethidine
An analgesic which can be injected in labour.

Placenta
The organ which feeds and supports the baby in the uterus, and removes waste products, also known as the afterbirth. It is about 20cm (8in) in diameter.

Posterior position
A term used to describe the baby facing away from the mother's spine in the uterus.

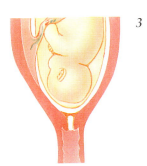

3

Pre-eclampsia
A condition which sometimes affects pregnant women, characterized by high blood-pressure, protein in the urine and oedema. This complication is checked for at every antenatal visit.

Progesterone
A hormone produced in early pregnancy. One of

its effects is to soften the smooth muscles, such as those of the internal organs.

Prolapse
A dropping down of the uterus because of lack of support.

Prostaglandins
Naturally occuring substances which, placed as a pessary in the vagina, soften and 'ripen' the cervix and stimulate labour. They occur in male semen, which is why making love can sometimes stimulate labour after the cervix has ripened.

Rectum
The end section of the large bowel, in which the faeces are stored. The baby's head can press on the rectum during birth, making you feel as though your bowels need emptying.

Surfactant
A substance which lines the inside surface of the lungs in order to prevent them collapsing on the outward breath.

Suture
Stitches.

Ultrasound
High-frequency sound waves which can produce a picture or scan of the baby.

Vacuum extraction
A suction pad on the baby's head used instead of forceps to help the baby out during birth.

Useful addresses

When writing for information, please enclose a stamped, addressed envelope.

Action on Smoking and Health
5-11 Mortimer Street
London
W1H 8BH

British Medical Acupuncture Society
67-9 Chancery Lane
London WC2 1AF

National Institute of Medical Herbalists
41 Hatherley Road
Winchester
Hants SO22 6RR

New Ways to Work
309 Upper Street
London
N1 2TY

Working Mothers' Association
23 Webbs Road
London
SW11 6RU

INDEX

A

Abdomen: changes in pregnancy 24, 63
  exercises for **80**
  massaging **106**
Aches *see* Pain
Acne 27
Alcohol, drinking 45
Allowances, maternity 52
Amniocentesis 122
Anaemia 118
Analgesics 122
Ankles: exercises for 75, **76**
  swollen 24, 119, 121
Antenatal care, choosing 112
Antenatal clinics:
  check-ups 113
  questions to ask 20-1
  time off for appointments 53
Anterior position 122
Antibodies 122
Anxieties in pregacy 12, 13, 15
Appetite: in pregnancy 48
  when breastfeeding 50
ARM *see* Artificial rupture of the membranes

Arms: exercises for **77**
  massaging **100, 103**
  puffy 119
Artificial rupture of the membranes 122
ASH (Action on Smoking and Health) 61
Assertiveness in pregnancy 20

B

Backache in pregnancy 63, 64-5, 118
Back exercises **76, 79, 80**
Back massage **100, 102**
  in labour **107**
Badminton 69
Bath: getting out 65
  massage in 107
Bathing: when pregnant 26
  after birth 32
Beauty plan 33
Bed, getting out of 65
Birth: active 122
  home 112
  natural 124
  positions for 85
  see also Labour
Bladder: changes in pregnancy 63, 114, 117
Blood pressure, changes in 63, 118

Body massage **102,** 104
Bras 40, **40, 41**
Braxton-Hicks contractions 122
Breastfeeding:
  and appetite 50
  positions for 66-7
  relaxing while 97
  see also Breasts
Breasts: changes in pregnancy 23, 24, 114
  massaging 26, 105
Breathing, deep 94
  in labour 95, 96-7
Breathlessness 30-1, 63, 118
Breech position 122
Buttocks, pain in 120

C

Caesareans 122
  and breastfeeding 66
  exercising after 86
Caffeine 45
Calcium requirements in pregnancy 42
Calorie requirements in pregnancy 42
Carrying babies 67
Cephalic 122
Cervix 122
Childminders 56
Cleansing creams 28

Clothes, maternity 34-9
  for hospital 41
Clumsiness 118-19
Coccyx 122
Coffee 45
Colostrum 24, 105, 117,
  123
Constipation 49, 119
Contractions 83, 123
  Braxton-Hicks 122
  see also Labour
Cramp 119
Curl ups (exercise) 78-9
Cycling 68, 69

D
Dancing 68, 69, 70
Day nurseries 56-7
Dental treatment 27
Diaphgram exercise **81**
Diet in pregnancy 42,
  43, 44, 46-7
Digestive system:
  changes in pregnancy
  63
Dizziness 119
Domino scheme 112, 123
Dreams, vivid 119-20

E
EDD see Expected day of
  delivery
Enemas 123
Engorgement 105, 123
Entonox 123
Epidural 123
Episiotomy 105, 123
Exercises 68, 74-5, 78-81
  postnatal 67, 86, **86-7**
  for relaxation 91
  warming-up 76-7
  in water 71
  yoga 72-3
Exfoliation 27
Expected day of delivery
  123
Eyes: changes in
  pregnancy 24
  shadows under 28
  puffiness round 28, 119

F
Face: exercises for **77**
  massaging **107**

and puffiness 28, 29, 119
Faintness 119
Falls in pregnancy 68
Fathers: ambivalent
  feelings of 16-17
  and sleeplessness 30, 31
  see also Massage
Fatty food 44, 47
Feet: exercises for 75, **76**
  swollen 24, 119
Fetal-heart monitor 123
Fetus, development of
  114-16
Fibre, dietary 44, 46
Fingers see Hands
Flatulence see Wind
Fluid retention 23, 119
Foetus see Fetus
Food see Appetite; Diet
Foundation, using 28
Fundus 123

G
Gingivitis 27
GP unit care 112
Grandparents 18
Grants, maternity 52
Gums, caring for 27

H
Haemorrhoids 120
Hair: caring for 29
  changes in pregnancy
  24
  loss of 24, 119
Hands: dry 23
  massaging **107**
  swollen 120
  tingling 120
Headaches 119
Head massage **100, 102-3**
Heart: changes in
  pregnancy 63
Heartburn 30-1, 49, 119
Herbal remedies 45
Home births 112
Hospitals: antenatal
  care 112
  clothes for 41
Housework 65, 69
Hunger see Appetite
Hypertension 123
Hypoallergenic products
  28

I
Indian cobbler position
  72, 73
Indigestion 30-1, 49, 119
Induction 123-4
Insomnia see
  Sleeplessness
Ironing 65
Iron tablets 44
  and constipation 49
Itchiness 119

J
Jealousy (in other
  children) 18, 19
Jogging 68, 69

L
Labour 82
  breathing techniques
  95, 96-7
  massage for 106, **106-7**
  onset of 117
  positions for 84-5
  relaxation in 91
  stages of 83
Lawn mowing 69
Leaking urine 67, 119
Legs: aching 118
  changes in muscles 63
  cramp in 119
  exercises for **76**
  massaging **100**, 104, **106**
  restless 120
Lifting: babies 67
  toddlers 65
Ligaments 63, 124
Linea nigra 24, 115
Lips, dry 28-9
Lungs 63
Lying down 65

M
Make-up in pregnancy
  28
Massage 98-9, 100, **100,**
  101
  for babies 108-9, **108,**
  109
  body **102**, 104
  in labour 106, **106-7**
Maternity allowances 52
Maternity clothes see
  Clothes

Maternity leave 52
Meconium 115, 124
Mineral supplements 44
Moisturizers 27
Mother's helps 57
Muscle tone, improving
 see Exercises

N

Nannies 57
Nappy changing 67
Nausea 119
 and food 48
Neck: exercises for **77**
 massaging **100, 103**
Nightmares 119-20
Nightwear **40**
 in hospital 41
Nipples *see* Breasts
Nose, stuffy 26, 120
Nosebleeds 120
Nurseries, day 56-7

O

Oedema 24, 119
Oxytocin 124

P

Pain: below bump 120
 between shoulders 120
 and massage 98-9
 pubic 120
 purpose of 82-3
 see also Backache
Part-time work 54-5
Pelvic-floor exercises
 67, **76, 78, 81**
Perineal massage 104-5
Perineum 124
Perms 29
Pethidine 124
Piles 120
Placenta 114, 124
Posterior position 124
Postnatal check-ups 113
Posture, good 64-5
Pre-eclampsia 124
Pregnancy 10-11
 anxieties in 12, 13, 15
 body changes in 63,
 114-17
Progesterone 124
Prolapse 124
Prostaglandins 124

Pubic pain 120
Puffiness 24, 28, 119

R

Rectum 124
Relaxation 90, 91
 when breastfeeding 97
 and breathing 94-5
 in labour 91
 whole-body 93
Ribcage: changes in 63
 pain in 120-1

S

Saliva, excess 121
Shampoos 29
Shared care 112
Shoes: casual 37
 formal 38
Shoulders: exercises
 for **77**
 massaging **100, 103**
 pain between 120
'Show', the 117
Sickness *see* Nausea
Sitting well 64
Skin: care of 27
 changes in 22-3, 24
 itchiness of 119
Sleeplessness in
 pregnancy 30, 121
Smoking, giving up 60-1
Snacks, healthy 50, 51
Soap 26
Spinal exercises **76, 79**
Sport 68, 69
Spots 27
Squash 69
Squatting exercise **78**
Stairs, climbing 65, 69
Standing well 64
Stomach *see* Abdomen
Stress, recognizing 90
Stretch marks 26
Support tights 23, 41
Surfactant 116, 124
Suture 124
Swaps, child 57
Sweating 24, 26
Swelling *see* Puffiness
Swimming 68, 69, 70

T

Tea 45

Teeth, caring for 27
Tennis 68, 69
Tension, recognizing 90
Thighs: massaging **100,**
 104, **106**
 pain in 120
Tidying up 65
Tights 23, 40-1
Tingling in hands 120
Tiredness 65, 121
Toddlers: coping with
 jealousy 18, 19
 lifting 65
Toners, skin 28
Trousers, maternity 35,
 36, **36, 37**

U

Ultrasound 124
Underwear 40, **40, 41**
Urine, leaking 67, 119
Uterus, changes in 63

V

Vacuum extraction 124
Vacuuming 65
Vagina: discharge from
 26, 121
 pressure in 120
Varicose veins 23, 121
Vernix 115, 116
Visual display units 53
Vitamin supplements
 44-5

W

Walking 69
Warming-up exercises
 76-7
Washing-up 65
Water exercises 71
 see also Swimming
Weight gain 43, 121
Wind 121
Womb *see* Uterus
Work: basic rights 52-3
 going back to 54
 stopping 53
Wrists: pain in 120
 swollen 24, 119
 tingling 120

Y

Yoga 68, 69, 72-3

Acknowledgments

Special thanks to Judith Schott, antenatal teacher and tutor, and Richard Worth, MA DPhil FRCS MRCOG, consultant obstetrician, for reading and commenting on the manuscript.

The publisher also wishes to thank the following for their help in the preparation of this book —

For illustrations: Gillie Newman and David Gifford

For taking part in the photography: Diane Garbutt, Gill Jones, Emily and Olivia, Michael Aristides

For permission to reproduce photographs in this book:
Front Jacket Photograph: Gibault/Jerrican.
3 Jacqui Farrow/Bubbles; **6** Anthea Sieveking/Network Photographers; **10** Loisjoy Thurston/Bubbles; **13** Jacqui Farrow/Bubbles; **14** Loisjoy Thurston/Bubbles; **16** Jacqui Farrow/Bubbles; **19** Anthea Sieveking/Network Photographers; **21** Jacqui Farrow/Bubbles; **22** Loisjoy Thurston/Bubbles; **25** Ron Sutherland; **33** Loisjoy Thurston/Bubbles; **34** Camera Press; **51** Loisjoy Thurston/Bubbles; **52** Jennie Woodcock; **55** Loisjoy Thurston/Bubbles; **60** Loisjoy Thurston/Bubbles; **62** Jacqui Farrow/Bubbles; **68** Jennie Woodcock/ Bubbles; **70** Sally and Richard Greenhill; **90** Loisjoy Thurston/ Bubbles; **95** Lupe Cunha; **97** Richard Yard/Bubbles; **105** Anthea Sieveking/Network Photographers; **110-111** Loisjoy Thurston/ Bubbles.

Special photography by Julie Fisher **4, 5, 8-9, 42, 45, 46, 49, 58-9, 72, 73, 74, 76, 77, 78, 79, 80, 81, 84, 85, 86, 87, 88-9, 92, 98, 100, 101, 102, 103, 106, 107, 108, 109.**